Relational Agents and Autonomy

OFF THE FENCE: MORALITY, POLITICS AND SOCIETY

Series editors: Arianne Shahvisi (Brighton and Sussex Medical School, UK), Peter West-Oram (Brighton and Sussex Medical School, UK) and Bob Brecher (University of Brighton, UK)

Publishing short, sharply-argued texts in applied moral and political philosophy, *Off the Fence* explores philosophy-in-use – at once rigorous, relevant and accessible. With an interdisciplinary focus, the series aims to tackle pressing real-world issues through clear and careful philosophical analysis, covering topics such as climate crisis, work, violence, consent, animal ethics, structural injustice, food and fascism. The series especially welcomes proposals from writers whose identities are under-represented in philosophy publishing, including those based in the Global South and those writing within non-Western philosophical traditions.

Title available in the series:

Kill Box: Military Drone Systems and Cultural Production, Alex Adams
Social Cohesion Contested, Dan Swain and Petr Urban
University in Crisis: From the Middle Ages to the University of Excellence, Michael Schapira
The Other Enlightenment: Self-Estrangement, Race, and Gender, Matthew Sharpe
Against Borders: Why the World Needs Free Movement of People, Alex Sager
The Troubles with Democracy, Jeff Noonan
The State and the Self: Identity and Identities, Maren Behrensen
Just Liberal Violence: Sweatshops, Torture, War, Michael Neu
Complicity: Criticism Between Collaboration and Commitment, Thomas Docherty
The Right of Necessity: Moral Cosmopolitanism and Global Poverty, Alejandra Mancilla

Relational Agents and Autonomy

A Lesson from Anorexia

Jacopo Condò

BLOOMSBURY ACADEMIC
LONDON • NEW YORK • OXFORD • NEW DELHI • SYDNEY

BLOOMSBURY ACADEMIC
Bloomsbury Publishing Plc, 50 Bedford Square, London, WC1B 3DP, UK
Bloomsbury Publishing Inc, 1359 Broadway, New York, NY 10018, USA
Bloomsbury Publishing Ireland, 29 Earlsfort Terrace, Dublin 2, D02 AY28, Ireland

BLOOMSBURY, BLOOMSBURY ACADEMIC and the Diana logo are trademarks of Bloomsbury Publishing Plc

First published in Great Britain 2026

A catalogue record for this book is available from the British Library.

A catalog record for this book is available from the Library of Congress.

ISBN: HB: 978-1-3506-1166-5
ePDF: 978-1-3506-1167-2
eBook: 978-1-3506-1168-9

Series: Off the Fence

Typeset by Newgen KnowledgeWorks Pvt. Ltd., Chennai, India

For product safety related questions contact productsafety@bloomsbury.com.

Contents

Introduction 1

1 Ethereal Anorexia 15

2 Anorexic Patients and Normative Gaps 37

3 The Separation between Autonomy and Reasons 51

4 Relational Autonomy and Monological Agents 71

5 The Conditions of the Exercise of Autonomy 91

6 Practices of Dialogical Responsibility 115

Conclusion 139

Glossary 143
Notes 147
Bibliography 189
Index 203

Introduction

Anorexia nervosa is a serious eating disorder characterized by extreme dietary restriction, an intense fear of weight gain and a distorted perception of body image. Treating anorexia is a serious challenge. Not only for its prognosis – 30 per cent of partial recovery and 20 per cent of treatment failure[1] – but because people with anorexia often, and very convincingly, deny having a problem. Many defend anorexia as a positive way of life, even as their 'true' identity, and refuse medical treatment. Tragically, this denial is a core feature of a condition with the highest mortality rate of any mental disorder (4–20 per cent)[2] and one that causes severe physical damage: heart and kidney failure, osteoporosis, amenorrhea and irreversible brain damage.[3]

One might think this isn't a real challenge. After all, the issue could be easily overcome by making treatment for anorexia compulsory (setting aside, for a moment, the impact of voluntariness on treatment outcomes). But this solution hits a major obstacle: under UK mental capacity law, most patients with anorexia are deemed capable of refusing treatment. Forcing treatment would thus violate basic human rights.

Conversely, some might argue that the solution is simple: respect the patient's right to autonomy. Yet this, too, leads to complications. Psychiatrists, patients in treatment and post-anorexics widely report that people with anorexia can lose the ability to reflect autonomously – even if they pass standard capacity assessments. Consequently, respecting their refusal may mean abandoning them to choices shaped by the disorder itself.

It is commonly assumed that individuals suffering from anorexia lack the ability to make fully autonomous decisions, especially when it comes to life-saving medical treatments. This assumption underpins current legal frameworks, such as the Mental Capacity Act 2005 (MCA), which adopts a value-neutral model of autonomy – focusing strictly on decision-making processes rather than the values or reasons behind the decisions themselves. This book critically examines the limitations of this value-neutral approach by closely exploring the real-life experiences and moral reasoning of individuals with anorexia, as well as insights from those who have recovered. Using concrete examples, I demonstrate how the MCA's approach often neglects the oppressive social and psychological conditions described by people with anorexia. Such oversight results in practical shortcomings and theoretical inconsistencies, particularly evident when anorexic patients refuse treatment.

My central argument is that these issues cannot be resolved without taking seriously what anorexia reveals about autonomy itself. Therefore, I propose an alternative, relational conception of autonomy – one that recognizes how our decisions and self-understanding are deeply influenced by our relationships, social contexts and cultural backgrounds. Adopting this relational perspective allows for a more nuanced and fine-grained understanding of autonomy, ultimately providing a better framework for respecting the rights and capacities of individuals with anorexia.

Aims and research questions

I examine the philosophical notion of autonomy through the lens of its medico-legal applications. In particular, I consider four key questions in this text: first, does value-neutrality ensure a non-discriminatory approach to decisional capacity? Second, can any conception of autonomy truly be value-neutral? Third, are irrational decisions necessarily non-autonomous? And fourth, why do value-neutral models of autonomy fail in the case of anorexic patients? To address these questions, I analyse the idea of the human agent, focusing especially on the concepts of *knowledge* and *self-knowledge*. This leads to a set of epistemological questions: Are agents epistemologically independent? Are reasons and values private? These questions are crucial for several reasons: they engage with central debates on autonomy within both liberal and feminist traditions; they respond to value-neutral concerns about non-discrimination and pluralism; they highlight the essential role of relationships, culture, history and language in shaping self-understanding; and, ultimately, they help lay the foundation for a more responsive and less oppressive approach to autonomy. In short, addressing these questions enables the development of a model of autonomy that is not only logically and legally coherent but also *applicable in real-life contexts and truly non-discriminatory*.

Values, reasons and the limits of value-neutrality

This book shows that value-neutrality fails to ensure a non-discriminatory approach to decisional capacity; that the notion of *private* values and reasons is both logically and practically unsustainable; and that the exercise of self-knowledge – and, more broadly, of autonomy – is deeply shaped by our relationships, social interactions, cultural backgrounds and historical contexts. Autonomy is not an isolated ability; it develops and functions within our connections to others and the world around us. These findings are significant for both medico-legal conceptions of autonomy and theories of relational autonomy. In the first case, they confirm that the model of autonomy embedded in the MCA is inadequate and discriminatory, and that it must be replaced by a conception of the agent that reflects our vulnerability, relationality and interdependence. More broadly, they reveal that key ideas within relational theories – such as interdependence, oppression and social embeddedness – cannot be meaningfully defended without adopting a radically relational view of agency, one that recognizes its *dialogical constitution*.

This work also contributes to our understanding of the decisional capacity of patients with anorexia and, more broadly, to research aimed at protecting and enhancing autonomy in individuals with mental disorders, disabilities or those living in conditions of oppression. I argue, first, that the perspectives of psychiatrists, patients with anorexia and post-anorexics on decisional capacity are systematically overlooked within the value-neutral framework. Second, I show that a genuinely responsive approach to treatment refusal must go beyond the functional criteria outlined in the MCA. It requires a more nuanced account of autonomy – one that incorporates relational conditions such as self-worth and dialogical accountability.

Finally, this study offers a new articulation of the work of Charles Taylor and Ludwig Wittgenstein within the context of medical ethics and practical philosophy. Their emphasis on the dialogical nature of language, reasons and values – combined with their practical and pluralist understanding of identity and freedom – creates the conceptual space for a more nuanced account of agency. This framework helps to overcome long-standing impasses in the autonomy debate and supports the development of a model of autonomy capable of recognizing impaired decisional capacity without relying on discriminatory solutions.

Value-neutrality and discrimination against anorexic patients

In medical ethics, the terms *mental capacity* and *decisional capacity* are often used interchangeably with *autonomy*,[4] referring to a patient's ability to make an informed, voluntary decision about their medical treatment. Under this view, autonomy plays a primarily defensive role: it protects individuals from external interference and secures their right to self-govern. According to both the MCA 2005 and the Convention on the Rights of Persons with Disabilities (CRPD, 2006), patients must be presumed capable of making medical decisions unless proven otherwise. When a person lacks mental capacity, decisions are made on the basis of their best interests.

The MCA adopts a value-neutral conception of autonomy, meaning that mental capacity assessments focus not on the content of the patient's values or reasons but on the decision-making process itself. As confirmed by the Court of Protection,[5] it is irrelevant whether a decision is based on irrational reasons – or even on no discernible reasons at all – so long as the patient can: (1) understand, (2) retain, (3) weigh relevant information, and (4) communicate a choice. If any of these four criteria are missing, the person is deemed non-autonomous.

As previous studies have shown,[6] the MCA's framework implies that most anorexic patients should be permitted to refuse life-saving treatment, since they typically meet all four of the required functional capacities. Yet this outcome clashes with psychiatric evidence, clinical experience and post-anorexic testimony. In response, the Court of Protection has consistently ruled that patients with anorexia lack capacity to refuse naso-gastric feeding – arguing that, *by definition*, they cannot make decisions about food. This conclusion, however, is deeply problematic. It morally discriminates against patients with anorexia based on their diagnosis and contradicts the core legal principles of the MCA and the CRPD: that autonomy must be presumed and cannot be denied solely on the basis of mental disorder. Epistemologically, it also forecloses any real inquiry into *why* or *how* anorexic patients may lack decisional capacity in the first place.

Simona Giordano has offered a thorough critique of the MCA's approach to eating disorders and decisional capacity,[7] highlighting the inadequacy and discriminatory nature of compulsory treatment based solely on psychiatric diagnosis. While I fully agree with her critique of how the MCA is applied to anorexic patients, I take issue with her proposed solution – namely, that patients who meet the MCA's procedural criteria should be allowed to refuse treatment.[8] Giordano argues that only a procedural assessment, like that endorsed by the MCA, can remain genuinely value-neutral. Any evaluation of the *content* of a patient's decision, she claims, risks being partial and unresponsive to their authentic values. Given the limits of *what we can legitimately know about others*, she concludes that we need not expand the criteria for autonomy: we should simply apply the MCA consistently and accept that anorexic patients who pass the assessment are fully autonomous and entitled to refuse life-saving treatment – a position she herself calls a 'brave claim'.[9]

Giordano's stance has the merit of aligning with the principles enshrined in the MCA and CRPD. Yet it remains at odds with the insights of clinicians, patients with anorexia and post-anorexics, as well as with empirical data on anorexia. Drawing on a broad set of sources – including interviews, autobiographies and clinical narratives – I argue that, in some cases,[10] anorexic patients *can* possess decisional capacity to refuse treatment. However, this does not make Giordano's conclusion any less hasty, based on questionable assumptions, or blind to key aspects of anorexics' treatment refusal. Despite its legal coherence, her solution proves no less problematic than the issue it seeks to resolve.

Autonomy and ordinary life

These complications are not limited to anorexic patients. Within medical ethics, the value-neutral approach to autonomy also presents serious challenges for individuals with depression, schizophrenia, bipolar disorder, DID, dementia and other conditions that affect a person's 'motivational set'. But the implications extend even further, reaching beyond medical ethics into broader contexts where multiculturalism, pluralism, oppression and vulnerability are central. Since the publication of Catriona Mackenzie and Natalie Stoljar's *Relational Autonomy* (2000),[11] the debate around autonomy has increasingly focused on reformulating the concept to address feminist critiques of agency and relationality. According to this line of thought, traditional accounts of autonomy rely on a mistaken image of the human being as independent, rational and atomistic. In contrast, feminist philosophy has shown that human beings are fundamentally *vulnerable*, *interdependent* and *socially*, *culturally* and *historically embedded*.[12]

Relational theorists argue that a viable notion of autonomy – one compatible with feminist critique and a non-idealist view of the agent – must account for the agent's relational embeddedness, the structural nature of oppression and the fundamental vulnerability and interdependence of human life. Autonomy, in this view, cannot be protected solely by shielding decision-making from external interference; it also requires responsiveness to the subtle and pervasive ways in which relational and cultural contexts can undermine agency. While all relational theorists share this core commitment, they differ in how they define the conditions under which autonomy is relationally impaired. 'Relational autonomy' is thus explicitly framed as an umbrella term – broad and internally diverse, encompassing perspectives that are sometimes deeply at odds.[13] This book maps that philosophical terrain, showing first that the key disagreements stem from divergent conceptions of the agent and second that only a narrow segment of this landscape provides a coherent and responsive framework for understanding the decisional capacity of anorexic patients.

Self-knowledge and dialogical conditions

This book contributes to the debate on relational autonomy by pursuing a path largely unexplored by other relational theorists. I develop a multi-layered defence of the dialogical and value-laden constitution of autonomy, focusing on the *dialogical structure of self-knowledge* and its implications for human agency. Drawing on the work of Charles Taylor and Ludwig Wittgenstein, I argue that self-knowledge is inherently dialogical: even the most *private* aspects of the self – such as identity and motivation – are relationally formed and expressed through language. In this sense, the idea of *direct, unmediated, private access* to one's own mental contents – assumed by defenders of value-neutrality as an *obvious* fact characterizing the human agent – turns out to be basically unsound, as well as being pragmatically inadequate. On the contrary, by acknowledging the dialogical nature of self-knowledge it becomes possible to offer a hermeneutically and logically sound account of autonomy and to lay the conceptual ground for understanding the role played by relational factors – such as dialogical answerability and self-regarding attitudes – in the *exercise* of autonomy. Although these elements are value-laden and require engagement with the *content* of the agent's motivational set, they do not entail the paternalism that defenders of value-neutrality fear.

Theoretical and medico-legal frameworks

This work is grounded in four key sets of factors: (1) the principles affirmed by the MCA and the CRPD – that autonomy must be presumed and that mental disorders do not automatically entail a lack of autonomy; (2) the concerns of value-neutral theorists about the potential for discrimination in value-laden conceptions of autonomy; (3) the testimonies of patients with anorexia and post-anorexic patients regarding their experiences of impaired autonomy in refusing treatment; and (4) the available empirical and epidemiological data on anorexia. My strategy is to address the failure of the value-neutral approach to anorexia while respecting these four commitments and avoiding any conclusion that would undermine them.

My central claim is that *value-neutrality cannot be upheld through a notion of the agent as epistemologically independent without violating these four principles.* If we accept the value-neutral position – that non-discrimination requires ignoring the reasons, values and content of a patient's decisions – we risk two equally problematic outcomes: discriminating against anorexic patients (as in the MCA's application) or abandoning them altogether (as in Giordano's 'brave claim'). Both approaches, I argue, are deeply unresponsive to empirical realities and the lived insights of people with anorexia and post-anorexics. Moreover, they rest on the denial of the value-laden and relational conditions essential for a coherent and practicable account of autonomy.

Value-ladenness, self-regarding attitudes and dialogical answerability

My findings fall into two broad categories: *critical* and *constructive*. The first half of the book concerns the first. Here, I offer an extensive analysis of the reasons underlying the failures of the value-neutral approach that allows me to highlight what *cannot* legitimately and reasonably be said about autonomy, specifically: that autonomy cannot coherently be understood as either value-neutral or as grounded solely in an agent's capacity to act on the basis of their private reasons and values. I come to this conclusion by analysing value-neutrality in the context of a wide range of data, insights, interviews, autobiographical accounts, as well as in terms of its legal and theoretical contradictions, highlighting the aspects of this approach that make it problematic.

The second half of the book is constructive. Staying within the boundaries of the four guiding factors outlined earlier, I develop a revised notion of autonomy by evaluating relational theories in light of the anorexia case and drawing on

Taylor and Wittgenstein's work on the dialogical constitution of knowledge. To avoid the pitfalls of Giordano's conclusion, I argue that all conceptions of autonomy are *necessarily* value-laden and normatively bounded – and that agency must be understood as *constitutively* relational. This requires a shift in perspective: value-neutrality is better conceived as an asymptote indicating a *tendency*, not an attainable state. Like the functional capacities enshrined in the MCA, values are not external to autonomy but an intrinsic aspect of how it is *exercised*.

To identify *which* value-laden conditions are relevant to the exercise of autonomy, I draw on the literature on *weak substantivism* – a view that connects autonomy with a set of dialogical attitudes, values and dispositions that neither predict nor directly constrain an agent's decisions. Its core claim is that the meaning of autonomy is inherently moral and cannot be reduced to purely value-neutral terms.[14] At a basic level, this means that autonomy is structurally tied to its own normative importance: recognizing its value is a prerequisite for exercising it. Autonomous agents understand themselves as *worthy* of taking responsibility for their lives and acting in accordance with their values and reasons. Without that sense of worth, agents are unable to engage their reasons as worth defending or expressing. From this perspective, *self-worth*[15] emerges as a key condition for exercising autonomy.[16] How can an act undertaken without such a background be considered an *act* at all?

Although self-worth is a self-regarding attitude, it is far from neutral – it is shaped by the value others accord to us, both directly and through social and cultural norms tied to gender, race, ethnicity, disability, religion or sexual orientation. It develops within relational contexts, which may or may not attribute worth justly. This relational understanding allows us to highlight aspects of the relation between oppression and autonomy that are undetectable from a value-neutral viewpoint: oppression erodes autonomy; oppressive circumstances institute a set of dialogical conditions that can erode the self-worth of those agents who are normatively devalued. Oppression is not a *sufficient* condition for heteronomy, but because social contexts deeply shape both the development and the viability of self-worth, special care is required when assessing autonomy in agents embedded in oppressive frameworks that diminish their perceived worth.

As I argue, the relational conditions for exercising autonomy do not lie solely in an agent's self-regarding attitudes but also in their disposition to engage dialogically with others. Autonomous agents are, to some degree, answerable to external critique and able to articulate their decisions in relation to their values and reasons. Agents do not develop their identity in isolation; they lack a private language and cannot fully understand themselves in solitude. Rather, identities, values and reasons take shape through interaction with, and against, others.

Agents who are not dialogically accountable or responsive to critique remain disconnected from the relational contexts where agency is formed, defended and expressed. Without this dialogical engagement, they are unable to show an *active*, reflective relation to their own reasons. By contrast, agents who are dialogically answerable demonstrate that their values are not simply internalized but actively held and articulated.

In practice, assessing dialogical answerability also requires acknowledging asymmetries of power. One party – the assessor – holds more authority, making it essential that they are genuinely committed to understanding the other's reasons, even when those reasons seem subversive, atypical or unsettling. This also entails close attention to what is expressed or shown by agents who feel excluded or oppressed within their relational context.

Normative structures cannot be entirely free from the risk of being oppressive. Still, it is surely possible to mitigate that risk. A focus on dialogical answerability aims to do precisely that. As Mackenzie writes, it 'provides grounds for criticizing social structures as unjust and reforming them, and it provides reasons for providing targeted social support and resources to scaffold the persons' capacities for self-governance'.[17]

Book structure

The book is divided into six chapters. The first, 'Ethereal anorexia', offers a multifaceted account of anorexia, drawing on a broad range of data to highlight the complexity of the phenomenon. I begin by reconstructing the psychiatric perspective, with particular attention to epidemiological data on incidence, prevalence and mortality. I then provide a brief historical overview, tracing the evolution of anorexia both psychiatrically and religiously. The chapter also explores anorexic and post-anorexic perspectives, guided by interviews conducted over more than fifteen years by Tan, Hope and colleagues. My aim here is twofold: first, to show how the psychiatric framework often overlooks the moral and identity-related dimensions of anorexia; and, second, to underscore that anorexics' views are deeply conflicted, often ambivalent, and resistant to reduction. Finally, I introduce two influential approaches – the familial and sociocultural perspectives – that interpret anorexia as an adaptive response to oppressive environments.

The second chapter, 'Anorexic patients and normative gaps', examines UK legislation on anorexics' refusal of treatment, focusing on the legal and ethical foundations of current practice. I highlight the shortcomings of the MCA (MCA), following Giordano's critique of how English law reduces, discriminates against and misrecognizes anorexic autonomy. While Giordano rightly challenges the law's assumptions about mental capacity in patients with anorexia, I extend this critique by drawing on recent research into body perception and eating behaviour. I argue that Giordano's 'brave claim' ultimately fails to resolve the dilemmas posed by anorexics' refusal of treatment, as it avoids rather than addresses the MCA's structural issues. Using Meyer's Double Axis theory, I show how Giordano's procedural solution, despite its moral focus, relies on an inadequate conception of values and cannot accommodate the nuanced insights of anorexics and post-anorexics. This chapter suggests that both the failures of current legal practice and Giordano's approach point to a deeper issue: the reductive, value-neutral conception of the agent. I argue for a re-evaluation of the role of values and reasons in autonomy.

The third chapter, 'The separation between autonomy and reasons', examines the rationale behind the separation of autonomy from reasons and values in both the MCA and Giordano's account. I outline two key views of reasons: internalism (adopted by both the MCA and Giordano) and externalism. While I acknowledge that externalism clashes with liberal commitments, I argue that internalism also fails to address the issues raised in the previous chapters regarding anorexics' reasoning and values. To move beyond the impasse between internalism and externalism, I draw on

Charles Taylor's notion of *background* and expose the monological structure underlying both the MCA and Giordano's approach.

The fourth chapter, 'Relational autonomy and monological agents', introduces and explores the notion of relational autonomy, tracing its development and key assumptions. I begin by outlining the feminist motivations for rethinking autonomy as a relational concept, distinguishing between procedural and substantive models, and reviewing major critiques of individualistic views. I argue that the divergences within the relational autonomy debate – particularly regarding oppression, vulnerability and embeddedness – stem largely from differing views of the relational agent. In turn, I show that causally relational accounts often retain a monological view of agency and remain tethered to proceduralism. Finally, I examine how proceduralist models, despite incorporating relational language, fail to adequately account for internalized oppression, false beliefs and adaptive preferences. This failure stems from their commitment to both a causal understanding of relationality and a fundamentally monological agent – a combination that ultimately contradicts the core insights of feminist and relational theory.

The fifth chapter, 'The conditions of the exercise of autonomy', builds on the previous analysis to map the philosophical terrain of relational autonomy and develop my own account, drawing on Taylor and Wittgenstein. I begin by arguing that any *coherent, viable,* value-neutral notion of autonomy must ultimately be *value-laden.* Autonomy is inherently normative, and value-neutrality should be treated not as a fully attainable quality but as an asymptotic ideal. I then offer a critique of the *epistemologically independent agent* – the idea that agents are *owners* of their reasons and values and have *unmediated* access to their mental contents. This view is epistemologically incoherent: it cannot explain how we commit mistakes in understanding ourselves, how mental contents are intelligible or how meaning arises before language. As Taylor and Wittgenstein argue, these capacities are rooted in shared practices of language, not private insight. Human understanding is relationally grounded: we learn to know ourselves because we first learn to speak with others. This perspective – which I refer to as *dialogical conception* – radically overturns monological epistemology: the primary form of human knowledge – that kind of knowledge that distinguishes human understanding from possible others' – is not private, but common; we learn to understand our own mental contents only because we first learn a language in which this possibility is realized. Autonomy, on this view, is not just relationally developed but relationally *exercised*. I close the chapter by identifying three conditions for the exercise of autonomy: (1) they concern the content of the agent's motivational set; (2) they are grounded in values that do not restrict the agent's outcomes; and (3) they are necessary but not sufficient. These conditions, I argue, align with *weak substantivism* – the view that links autonomy with dialogical dispositions and attitudes, without prescribing what agents must choose.

The sixth and final chapter, 'Practices of dialogical responsibility', applies the dialogical conception of autonomy developed earlier to the ethical-legal dilemmas explored in Chapter 2. I begin by challenging the liberal notion of intervention. From a monological perspective, autonomy is treated as a private property to be protected from all external interference, including supportive scaffolding. But if relational interactions are constitutive of agency, then intervention can be understood as a form of support – a practice of *relational responsibility* aimed at protecting and enhancing autonomy. I then articulate how relational autonomy – particularly self-regarding attitudes and dialogical answerability – should inform the assessment of mental capacity in anorexic patients who refuse treatment. If self-worth is constitutive of autonomy, a decision cannot be considered autonomous if the agent does not see herself as worthy of making it. Applied to anorexia, this means that configurations of self-worth, self-trust and self-respect – shaped by the egosyntonic traits of the disorder – must be assessed case by case. Egosyntonic self-worth should not automatically disqualify a patient's decision, but its defensibility must be evaluated through the lens of dialogical answerability.

To clarify this, I analyse two paradigmatic cases: a patient who has never received treatment and one with severe and enduring anorexia (SEAN). In the first case, I argue that while there is no universal model for assessing dialogical answerability, such patients typically come to reject anorexia only through treatment and the support of others. Thus, patients who have never been treated should not be permitted to refuse life-saving treatment. SEAN patients present a more complex picture. They may have deeper insight into their condition and a more reasoned basis for refusing treatment. While their motives may be painful, they can be coherent in light of their values, histories and lived experiences. Still, SEAN is neither terminal nor untreatable – recovery remains possible, and treatments are evolving. Even so, I argue that these considerations alone cannot override their refusal. I conclude by stressing two key points for future research and clinical practice. First, we need a better understanding of the roles that self-trust and self-respect play in the onset, persistence and treatment of anorexia. Second, intervention should not be limited to life-threatening scenarios: early intervention remains the most effective strategy we have.

1

Ethereal Anorexia

The challenge presented by anorexia is real and profound. It affects not just patients but families, communities and, more broadly, the ethical and legal frameworks that underpin society. This issue is not restricted solely to anorexia or those closely involved. Rather, as I aim to demonstrate, it exposes deep tensions within our society's normative structure. It violently puts in crisis the hierarchy of the values embraced by liberal societies and, ultimately, the notion itself of autonomy and individuality. Allow me to expose the reason why this is the case.

As mentioned, UK law typically finds anorexic patients mentally competent to refuse treatment. Yet, in practice, courts often approve compulsory treatment even after a positive capacity assessment. I'll return later to the medical, ethical and legal aspects of this. For now, the key point is this: such exceptions are unacceptable. By forcing treatment despite acknowledged competence, the system discriminates against anorexic patients – and reveals its own limits.

Let me be clear: I'm not claiming patients with anorexia should or shouldn't be deemed competent. My point is that the current model for assessing mental capacity fails to capture the complexity of anorexic autonomy. And this failure can't be solved without rethinking *autonomy* from the ground up. If we want to avoid rushed, harmful solutions and obtain a better understanding of how mental capacity can shift in certain – but not extraordinary – conditions, we must reconsider what it means to be autonomous and face the consequences of doing so.

That's where my argument is headed. But first, we need to clarify the core issues – anorexia and mental capacity legislation. These are complex topics, and I'll dedicate a full chapter to each. Let's begin with anorexia.

The psychiatric perspective and some data

According to the *International Classification of Diseases, ICD-10* and the *Diagnostic and Statistical Manual of Mental Disorders, DSM-V*, the main characteristic of anorexia is deliberate weight loss – below 85 per cent of that expected[1] – achieved through severe food restriction and compensatory practices such as self-induced vomiting, excessive physical exercise and the use of laxatives and appetite suppressants. Anorexia is marked by an intense fear of gaining weight and a distorted perception of body shape and size. Most patients also experience anxiety, depression, mood and personality disorders, low self-esteem, guilt, perfectionism and self-harming or compulsive behaviours.[2]

Unlike many other mental disorders, anorexia has a well-defined clinical profile, making diagnosis relatively straightforward.[3] There's no conclusive evidence that any single treatment is superior, but early intervention tends to be more effective.[4] In recent years, treatment outcomes – especially relapse rates and weight recovery in adolescents – have improved.[5] Treatment usually follows three phases: weight restoration, psychological therapy and management of behaviours and thoughts that maintain the disorder.[6] The high mortality rate is mainly due to suicide and heart failure.[7]

Current statistics place anorexia's prevalence between 0.9 per cent and 4.3 per cent[8] mainly in Western and Westernized[9] countries.[10] It primarily affects young women aged fifteen to nineteen[11] and is more common in fields where thinness is idealized, such as modelling and dance.[12] Still, epidemiological data remain limited due to the difficulty of long-term population screening, social stigma and patients' reluctance to seek help.[13]

The causes of anorexia are unknown.[14] Twin studies have shown that the concordance rate of anorexia is higher among monozygotic twins (44 per cent) than dizygotic (12.5 per cent), suggesting genetic factors in the onset of the disorder.[15] Contextual components, especially social, cultural and familial, are also considered significant.[16] Still, some scholars insist that anorexia is not a simple social or familial effect but a personal and moral way in which the individual copes with the environment.[17]

The first medical report of anorexia – described as a 'nervous consumption' – was made by the English physician Richard Morton in 1689,[18] but the appearance of the term 'anorexia nervosa' dates back only to October 1873 with the publication of two articles written respectively by Ernest-Charles Lasègue and William Withey Gull.[19] In 1914 the German pathologist Morris Simmonds found damage in the pituitary glands of some patients with anorexia, and for more than twenty years the disorder was associated with 'Simmonds' disease' or 'pituitary cachexia' (a syndrome ascribed to damage of the hypophysis).[20] Between 1945 and 1960 psychoanalytic studies framed anorexia as rooted in unconscious fears of oral incorporation.[21] A major shift came with Hilde Bruch's work, which redefined anorexia as a disorder marked by low self-esteem, distorted body image and the rigid pursuit of thinness.[22] In 1983, the death of singer and drummer Karen Carpenter at age thirty-two from heart failure caused by anorexia brought widespread public attention to eating disorders.

It's worth noting that for centuries in Europe, self-starvation wasn't seen as pathological but as part of the ascetic ideal in religious life. One of the earliest examples appears in the bodily purification practices of the Hellenistic Era. The first documented death by self-starvation dates to 383 AD, when a Roman woman died following the ascetic teachings of St Jerome.[23] In the Middle Ages, *inedia prodigiosa* – now known as *anorexia mirabilis* – described women and girls who 'miraculously' fasted in devotion to divine purity.[24] Saint Catherine of Siena (1347–1380) saw starvation as a path to God,[25] while Saint Theresa of Avila fasted and used olive twigs to induce vomiting.[26] In Victorian England, gender norms idealized women as thin, ethereal, asexual and self-disciplined – an aesthetic some scholars argue helped create the cultural conditions for the rise of anorexia.[27]

Anorexic perspectives

Even when people with anorexia fully understand the nature of the disorder and the risks to their health, they often resist the very treatments that could save their lives. Jacinta Tan, Tony Hope and colleagues have explored this refusal in depth, showing that issues of identity and authenticity are central.[28] Their work, developed in collaboration with patients and families through extensive interviews, offers very valuable insight into how people with anorexia perceive their condition.

The quotes from interviews conducted by researchers such as Tan, Hope and colleagues do not aim to present a definitive 'anorexic viewpoint'. Rather, my selection of these accounts aims to highlight that, although these views differ and resist reduction to a single narrative, they all share a concern with identity and morality, aspects often overlooked in psychiatric approaches. Medical definitions focus on observable behaviours – deliberate weight loss, compensatory practices, fear of weight gain – but tend to ignore the deeper personal and moral meaning these behaviours hold for the individual. Many people with anorexia see the disorder as deeply tied to their identity and decision-making capacity, and often view its impact as central and even positive in their lives.

I divide my discussion of anorexics' perspectives on anorexia into four groups: (A) egosyntonicity, (B) divided self, (C) positive and (D) negative relations with anorexia. In the first two groups I have selected interviews that focus on the relation between identity and anorexia. In (A) anorexia is considered an integral and essential part of the self, while in (B) it is experienced as a distinct entity that conflicts and usurps the self. In the last two groups I have chosen the interviews that underline how anorexia can be considered in (C) positive and (D) negative terms.

(A) It is quite common for people with anorexia, especially when they are still not decisively underweight, to experience anorexia as their authentic self or as part of a single integrated self:

Interviewer: What does your anorexia nervosa mean to you?
Participant A: It is quite a lot. It feels like my identity now, and it feels like … I suppose I worry that people don't know, they don't know the real me.[29]
Interviewer: Let's say you've got to this point, and someone said they could have a magic wand and there wouldn't be anorexia any more.
Participant I: I couldn't
Interviewer: You couldn't.

Participant I: It's just a part of me now.

Interviewer: Right. So it feels like you'd be losing a part of you.

Participant I: Because it was my identity.[30]

Participant 17: Quite often, people with anorexia, they don't say, 'I have anorexia', they say 'I am anorexic'. And I think that's kind of, that explains it really, that shows what it is, people BECOME anorexic, they, and then they start saying, 'I am anorexic', and it's this kind of, it becomes who you are, it defines who you are, as opposed to just an illness that you have.[31]

Participant A highlights how anorexia can be experienced as the true self. She fears others won't understand who she really is – echoing Participant I's view that she and her anorexia are inseparable. Participant 17 adds that anorexia isn't just an illness but something so deeply embedded that changing it would mean losing oneself. For patients with egosyntonic anorexia, accepting treatment is especially painful, as it feels like a fundamental loss of identity:

Participant C: I could be happy [without anorexia] – but it would be a completely different me, it would be a completely different way of thinking, because I don't think I could be the person I want to be, at the moment, without anorexia, because it's a part of it.[32]

Participant 18: If [anorexia] almost does become part of you and so in order to get it out of you I think you do have to kind of hurt you in the process, I think it's almost inevitable.[33]

(B) However, egosyntonicity represents only one phase or aspect of the experience of anorexia. Many patients feel ambivalent about their identification with anorexia. Especially among those in treatment, anorexia is sometimes seen as a separate entity that conflicts with the self. These patients often view the ability to distinguish between the 'anorexic' self and the 'real' self as a crucial – though fragile – achievement.

Participant 36: It feels like there's two of you inside, like there's another half of you, which is my anorexia and then there's the real K [own name], the real me, the logic part of me and it's a constant battle between the two … So there's always the real me still there because, well, if the real me wasn't there, then I'd be dead, because the real me is what I use to fight against it and to motivate me to want to beat it and get well. I truly believe that, that if there wasn't any me left, if there was none of me inside of me then I would have let it kill me by now. [The idea of the real me] is very helpful. If I didn't have that, then – I mean, I know people who haven't got that, and they're very much stuck in their recovery, perhaps won't ever recover, yet I know people who have recovered who, like me, very know the difference between the two. I definitely know the difference between the two.[34]

Participant 38: I don't think it [anorexia] does feel alien. I think it is part, it feels like it's part of me, but I like to now believe that it's not part of me, it's just something else that I can get out and it's just some other thing … I think with it being part of me, I still do feel it is part of me to some degree, and I, that makes me still want to hold on to it … but then at the same time I can see that I don't want it to be part of me and the only way to get rid of it is to really hate it and be really angry with it and get it way from me.[35]

Participant 36 identifies her real self with logical thinking, in contrast to anorexia – the 'other' half she believes would lead her to death. Participant 38, by contrast, doesn't see anorexia as separate from herself, yet she resists this identification and struggles to break away from it. Both participants place strong value on being able to distinguish between the anorexic and the true self. It's common for patients to feel one part of the self as more dominant depending on their weight:

Participant 36: When it takes control, particularly when I'm at a very low weight, its voice if you like is loud, very, very loud, and I can't, the real me can't battle against it … When I start to get better and put on weight and get well, then the real me gets stronger and so it goes down, and then I'm like 75/25, 50/50, and I'm hoping eventually 100/nothing.[36]

The internal conflict in anorexia can be overwhelming, making it hard for patients to recognize or express what they truly feel. The tension between an intense fear of food and the desire to recover can become so heavy that it leads some to stop resisting and continue self-starving.

Participant 20: So I didn't really want treatment, but then there's this little voice deep down inside, which is kind of the complex part, that's saying 'you know you do want treatment really', but then there's this kind of overriding big THING which is just like 'no, you're FAT' (laughs), 'you don't need to put on weight!'[37]

Rachel: I would describe anorexia as a little person in the back of your head screaming at you. It is a little person that tells you that you want to be alone, that you don't need friends, that you don't need family, that you need to eat as little as possible, and you need to exercise this certain amount. And it's this little thing that puts demands on you and says that 'you will be accepted. You are the winner or you're the best. You are better than anyone or anything if you don't eat'. And it is this little voice that is trying to kill you. But you don't see it. I don't see it. I don't see this voice as killing me sometimes. I see it as my best friend. So in some ways it's a security blanket. It's my best friend, but my best friend is trying to kill me.[38]

The loss of control experienced by people with anorexia can be seen as inscribed in a wider issue about control. Paradoxically, for most people experiencing anorexia, self-starving is a way of gaining self-control.

Participant D: I think [anorexia] begins with a need to control when individuals feel that various areas of their life are out of control, and they're not happy about other areas of their lives, and so they look for another way to feel in control, to feel happiness, and a way you can guarantee it is by food, by weight, by exercise.[39]

Interviewer: You mentioned that anorexia is a symptom of something else. What is it a symptom of for you?

Rachel: For me, I think my whole life I wanted control. And I want sameness and control and an identity and to feel accepted in some way. And I think at some point my anorexia became my identity.[40]

(C) Anorexia has proper positive aspects, such as providing a sense of self-control or serving as a distraction from other problems. Since the late 1990s,[41] pro-anorexia websites, blogs, forums and social media pages have emerged to promote these perceived benefits.

These spaces share what are colloquially known as *thinspirations* – images, songs and videos intended to promote extreme thinness – as well as weight-loss stories and tips on severe dieting, drugs and exercise.[42] Pro-ana communities typically don't view anorexia as a disorder but as a lifestyle built on self-control and discipline.

> We [anorexics] are 'thrivers'! We thrive upon challenge, upon competition, upon the raw stimulation of life, keenness of our senses, strength and artistry in our bodies, alertness and clarity in our minds. We thrive upon the fact that while all religions, philosophies, ideologies upon the earth extol the virtues of self-control and self-government, our path alone holds the key to unlock the most secret chambers of these mysteries in something so seemingly simple as an empty plate, in something so seemingly shallow as a desire to be thin.[43]

The anonymous context of the internet and the comfort offered by friendly communities support pro-ana members in expressing their view of anorexia in a blameless manner that is difficult to find in interviews.[44] Notwithstanding that, even in the formal context of interviews, appreciation of the positivity of anorexia is not uncommon:

Participant F: It [anorexia] takes control of you, but it can also feel very safe. It's a very confusing illness, because at the moment it's probably got a lot of control over me, in certain ways, and I just want to get away from it, I'm just sick and tired and I'm exhausted, but then it kind of protects you as well, I think, from coping with other things.[45]

Participant 16: There's this little emotion that seems to accompany being thin, and I can't it, I can't really, I don't really have the language to explain it, it's a very um, but you sort of, you have this sort of, I don't know, sort of like serenity and calm. You know you feel very, very calm and comfortable and sort of I guess safe, a mixture of all those sort of things. And sort of security and sort of just RIGHTEOUSNESS as if this is the right thing … it's a very nice way to feel.[46]

The appreciation of anorexia as something beneficial is not limited to the first stages of the disorder. In some cases, people continue to praise the benefits of anorexia even in its later stages and despite serious physical risks.

Participant D: I remember getting some tests back saying how my liver was really damaged and all this, and I thought it was really rather good! I can't imagine that I thought it, it felt like really quite an accomplishment! … I'd just done something that I knew hardly anyone else could do … I can remember when I had difficulty walking upstairs, or I had such pain bending down, at the back of my legs, and I loved it, I used to bend down as much as I could to feel the pain! And I felt so in control.[47]

(D) Even if some people begin to resist anorexia only after recovery, there are moments in every anorexic history when the perceived benefits of self-starvation and compensatory behaviours turn into burdens. The sense of control anorexia once provided flips into a terrifying loss of control. Suppressed thoughts resurface, often more forcefully than before. In these moments, anorexia is linked to loss of control, self-punishment, guilt and low self-esteem.

Participant 21: I think you feel you can control um, have extra control in your life by controlling what food you eat very, very strictly but in the end it doesn't end up you controlling it, it's kind of more it controlling you because I found in the end um, I found in the end that if I had wanted to make any choice, different choices that I couldn't do it so it wasn't, it wasn't really my own choice any more.[48]

Participant 17: [Anorexia] is a prison, it's not just about food, it's about life I think 'cos I find that it's made me want to control everything.[49]

Participant F: It kind of protects you as well, I think, from coping with other things. It just distracts you the whole time. Basically punishing you all day long, bullying you about something. It just fills your mind. It distracts you so completely about things you don't want to think about, to lose that is quite scary.[50]

Janet: I don't feel I deserve [to eat]. I don't feel I deserve nice clothes. When my sister died I thought it should have been me.[51]

Anorexia becomes deeply problematic for those who experience it. Social life often breaks down because it is hard to maintain strict eating rules and compensatory behaviours around others. Starvation and these practices weaken the heart, kidneys, bones and stomach. A key issue is the conflict between wanting to avoid anorexia's physical and social consequences and the fear of gaining weight. For some, this conflict fades: they come to believe it's impossible to stop, especially due to the intense, unbearable emotions food provokes.

Participant 21: Well I always THOUGHT that I could, like before I tried it I thought all the time well I could easily eat more and stop this if I wanted. But when I came to try to do that I couldn't.[52]

Participant 13: When I was lying in the hospital my mum would bring over a bowl of melon and say 'Melon OK, it's just water' … I'd thinking, 'oh I really want to eat that, I want to eat, I just want to eat'. … And then when it came to it, my hands would start shaking and I'd just want to throw it across the room, I just couldn't do it, no matter how hard I tried I just couldn't physically do it … I don't even know what was stopping me, it was obviously the anorexia but my thought just changed, like one minute I would, and the next minute I just went 'NO' I couldn't do it, at all.[53]

Patients overwhelmed by anorexia often describe it as a separate entity that takes over their lives. Yet their estrangement from it is complex and ambivalent. On the one hand, they see anorexia as alien and harmful; on the other, they feel trapped by it, defend their behaviours, or deny being ill. For many, anorexia is not just central to their life; it's seen as part of who they are.

People with anorexia express conflicting, ambiguous and shifting views about the disorder. Still, two axes can help map these perspectives: the unified–divided-self axis and the positive–negative evaluation axis. Most anorexic viewpoints fall somewhere along these spectrums, often reflecting internal contradictions. Positive views are more common in early stages, while divided-negative and unified-negative views tend to emerge during treatment. Of these, only the divided-negative stance seems to mark a possible transition towards recovery.

Post-anorexic perspectives

Generally, post-anorexics don't feel they have *completely* recovered from anorexia.[54] Some retain a subtle identification with anorexia, while others believe that anorexia is still present in their life – even if not in a harmful manner.[55] Almost every post-anorexic considers their history as one in which anorexia is fundamental for their self-understanding.

Anne: If you have something that is a part of your personality, it's a part of you, it's got to be … it's in your blueprint somewhere … Otherwise you wouldn't have taken it onboard in the first place.[56]

Participant 31: [Anorexia is] quite an important factor in sculpting who I am. I am not really it anymore, but what it's left behind has sort of made me.[57]

Anorexia often persists in two ways. First, as a lingering temptation – something that remains present even after recovery. Post-anorexics are typically aware of the risk of relapse and often describe anorexia using the language of addiction.

Jane: There's always going to be warning bells, the same as an alcoholic will still get those triggers.[58]

Naomi: I still am always cautious that I could fall into the trap again … in the same way that an alcoholic is always an alcoholic.[59]

Second, it persists as a crucial experience that has shaped post-anorexic identity, values and capacities.

Naomi: It's like anorexia is always in there, it's part of who I am, it's part of my fabric, it's part of what I value, it's part of what I think of my morals, my ethics, all those type of things that flavour who I am.[60]

Susan: That experience that you've had also definitely shape you … Being more empathetic and more accepting of other people … I would like to stay more in touch with it actually.[61]

The first-person experience of anorexia often contrasts with the psychiatric view, especially in terms of values and lived experience. Both anorexic and post-anorexic individuals see anorexia as more than a disorder – they describe it as deeply tied to moral and identity issues that the medical model fails to capture.[62] In *The Anorexic Self*, Paula Saukko describes these identity struggles as a dialogue between conflicting social expectations.[63] She argues that the split between a 'true' and a 'false' (anorexic) self stems directly from the dominance of the psychiatric narrative on anorexia:

> The aim of my autoethnography is … to address the fact that my experience [of anorexia] is only accessible to me through the discourses on eating disorders, which I have both violently resisted and incorporated into my self-image. I seek to illuminate, from the inside out, the occasionally illuminative but also limiting and misguiding effects that psychiatric and public discourses on anorexia had for my treatment and self-understanding.[64]

Saukko makes a key claim: recognition of anorexia is grounded in psychiatric and public discourses that fail to fully capture the anorexic experience. What's missing, she argues, are the moral and personal dimensions that shape how anorexia is lived.

> The anorexic experience is often driven by a desire to create a 'new', better self …, as well as to destroy an unacceptable self.[65]

From her perspective, anorexic resistance is not just a symptom but a response to the 'monologue' of medical and public narratives. While these frameworks help shape how anorexia is understood, they a priori exclude the possibility that anorexics' voices are meaningful. Seeing people with anorexia only as victims of a disorder or as having a 'false' self reduces the depth of their claims and experiences. Saukko links this exclusion to the rise of pro-ana communities: feeling misunderstood and misrepresented, many turn to spaces that allow them to express their experience more freely. She argues that the dominant view of pro-ana communities should be reconsidered:

> Participants in the pro-ana communities … define starving in more ambivalent and aspirational terms and view it as a response to deep-seated or serious life disturbance … They should not be denounced as dangerous, but they should not be romanticized as resistance either.[66]
>
> Analyses of posts on pro-ana Web sites have revealed that anorexics often experience their condition as simultaneously empowering and damaging.[67]

Whether these spaces are harmful remains a thorny issue.[68] Still, beyond serving as sources of data, pro-ana communities offer a place where anorexia is expressed as both empowering *and* destructive, positive *and* negative.

Both people with anorexia and post-anorexics affirm that anorexia involves issues far beyond the clinical definition – issues central to moral identity and self-understanding. Many post-anorexics maintain a subtle connection to anorexia and rarely view recovery as complete. Anorexia is deeply tied to autonomy, identity and morality, and many aspects of it – especially those seen as positive – are ignored in medical discourse. Sociological and feminist approaches help fill this gap, focusing on relational dynamics and exploring what psychiatric perspectives leave out. These will be explored in the next section.

Perspectives on family relationships

Social, cultural and familial factors are widely recognized as relevant to the development of eating disorders.[69] Anorexia often affects young women raised in families marked by contradictory values and weak emotional bonds.[70] Sociological and feminist scholars agree that anorexia cannot be fully understood without accounting for these contexts, and some go further, arguing that such factors can explain the disorder entirely. In these accounts, anorexia is seen as an *expression* of social, cultural or familial dynamics.

While epidemiological data on anorexia's prevalence and incidence remain somewhat unreliable – due to the challenges of long-term population screening – scholars have made significant efforts to improve accuracy. Anna Goodman, Amy Heshmati and Ilona Koupil, for example, tracked over 2 million Swedish individuals born between 1973 and 1998 over four years,[71] refining earlier British and Swedish studies.[72] Their findings show that anorexia occurs more often in families with high educational levels, while parental income and social class appear statistically irrelevant.[73]

This challenges the earlier approach to anorexia – such as those of Bruch and Palazzoli – which linked anorexia to the pressures of upper-class families.[74] Rather than being limited to specific social groups, anorexia appears influenced by family education levels, likely due to the cultural value placed on academic achievement. This aligns with other research showing that parental expectations and social comparison contribute to feelings of frustration and dissatisfaction with one's appearance – factors associated with increased eating disorder risk.

Goodman et al. suggest that the link between anorexia and family education levels reflects the cultural value placed on education. This view aligns with other studies on anorexics' families, which highlight the role of parental expectations and familial pressure.[75] Emphasis on academic and social success – and the social comparison that comes with it – can foster frustration and dissatisfaction with one's appearance, both known risk factors for eating disorders.[76] Goodman et al. also confirm the statistical significance of emotional neglect, childhood sexual abuse and parental perfectionism in anorexia's development.[77] Interestingly, despite psychiatry's focus on weight and shape control, a family or personal history of dieting appears to be a less significant predictor.

Mara Selvini Palazzoli's pioneering research highlights how parents of people with anorexia often deny responsibility for negative dynamics within the family.[78] She also points to a key theme echoed in feminist approaches: daughters typically receive mixed messages about their roles. They're expected to be both self-sacrificing caregivers and independent, high-achieving individuals.

While clinical studies tend to be cautious in interpreting this data, they generally present anorexia as a response to family-related pressures. Research suggests it functions as a defensive or maladaptive strategy to cope with the conflicting demands of a high-pressure, emotionally unsupportive environment – where control, comparison and expectations are constant. In this context, anorexia becomes a way to assert and gain self-control.[79]

Although findings from family studies are statistically consistent, they remain within the realm of probability, not causation. Research on anorexia is still limited – due to patients' reluctance to seek help, the need for long-term screening and a lack of comprehensive data. Moreover, establishing a causal link between family context and anorexia is inherently problematic. It's nearly impossible to isolate specific causal factors from the complex web of influences surrounding them.

Even identifying the effects of these presumed causes is difficult, as similar factors may lead to entirely different disorders – such as unipolar depression, bipolar disorder or anxiety.[80] Gregory Bateson, for instance, suggested in *Steps to an Ecology of Mind* that conflicting family expectations (or 'double binds') are necessary for developing schizophrenia.[81] In short, while acknowledging the role of family factors may be helpful for prevention and therapy, it does not offer proof of a causal relationship with anorexia.

Feminist studies frame anorexia as a gendered issue. In her analysis of female vampire figures and their link to anorexia, Domínguez-Rué explores how Western culture – especially in the Victorian era – idealized women 'as angelic beings, [while] they are simultaneously feared as a sexually voracious monster'.[82] The Victorian ideal of 'True Womanhood' was tied to the image of a fragile, delicate body, symbolizing spiritual (as opposed to carnal or masculine) nature. In contrast, a fuller female body and visible appetite were linked to uncontrolled sexuality and 'unnatural' desire. The 'True Woman' was expected to control her hunger and behaviour, suppressing her 'diabolic' impulses to assume the form of the ethereal woman. Female hunger thus became a metaphor for dangerous, transgressive desire – opposed to the traditionally masculine traits of self-control, willpower and intellect.

In one of the most representative texts in this regard, *Unbearable Weight: Feminism, Western Culture, and the Body*, Susan Bordo writes:

> The mythology/ideology of the devouring, insatiable female … is the image of her female self the anorexic has internalized. … Hungering, voracious, extravagantly and excessively needful, without restraint, always wanting too much affection, reassurance, emotional and sexual contact, and attention. … Anorexia nervosa … can be seen at least in part a defence against the 'femaleness' of the body and a punishment of its desires. Those desires have frequently been culturally represented through the metaphor of female appetite. The extremes to which the anorexic takes the denial of appetite (that is, to the point of starvation) suggest the dualistic nature of her construction of reality: she transcends body totally, becoming pure 'male' will, *or* she capitulates utterly to the degraded female body and its disgusting hungers.[83]

Western and Westernized societies place high value on women's ability to control and transcend the body. Drawing on Foucault, Bordo interprets social practices like framing female appetite as inappropriate as tools of bodily discipline, as a form of control of individuals, underlining how the development of identities is unavoidably 'in the grip' of cultural practices.[84] She argues that women, more than men, are subject to intense cultural pressure around body and food. Thinness is idealized, while the dominant cultural narrative associates the female body with a natural inclination to disorganization and indiscipline.

Rationality is coded as masculine – linked to self-control and discipline – while women are associated with emotional excess and uncontrolled appetite. Within this framework, the only socially accepted path for women to gain moral and social recognition is through mastering their body and appetite (their *femininity*, in terms of the social narration) in order to achieve those capacities that are 'naturally' the property of men.

As Bordo argues, women – whether they conform to or reject these gender norms – inevitably engage in a struggle over their bodies, centred on appetite and control. The 'alien self' felt by people with anorexia, she suggests, isn't simply a symptom of illness but a culturally shaped experience of the very female body that conflicts with the culturally dominant male ideals:

> The anorexic's *other* self – the self of the uncontrollable appetites, the impurities and taints, the flabby will and tendency to mental torpor – is the body ... But it is also (and here the anorexic's associations are surely in the mainstream of Western culture) the *female* self. These two selves are perceived as at constant war. But it is clear that it is the male side – with its associated values of greater spirituality, higher intellectuality, strength of will – that is being expressed and developed in the anorexic syndrome.[85]

Bordo takes a 'hard'[86] explicative approach towards the cultural aspects of anorexia, arguing that people with anorexia *surely* associate femininity with the unmanageable aspects of the body because this link is deeply embedded in Western culture. If the female body is culturally framed as impure, unstable and indolent, *it is clear* that anorexia should be considered a way of achieving the male-coded ideals of willpower and intellect.

According to Bordo, anorexia is less about conforming to feminine beauty standards and more about claiming the self-discipline and control traditionally reserved for men. Through self-starvation, individuals manage the 'unmanageable' female body and transcend their cultural role, aligning their identity with the male ideal of pure will. In line with familial theories, Bordo concludes that anorexia functions as an adaptive strategy to gain control in a hostile environment.

As we've seen, Saukko – like Bordo – emphasizes the role of gendered structures in the development of anorexia, highlighting the contradictory position assigned to women in Western culture.

> Both psychiatry and feminism concluded that anorexia articulates women's (feminine) inability to live up to the ideal, healthy (masculine) autonomous

> or independent self … Perfectionism is the only available strategy for attaining success for many women, who are pushed to extreme trying by the structural imperative, sugarcoated by the ideology of equal opportunities, that tells women and blacks that they can succeed as well as white men if they just try hard enough.[87]

But it's not only gender roles that create the conditions for anorexia; Western societies also promote behaviours closely tied to the disorder, such as extreme perfectionism and self-control. According to Saukko, the anorexic experience of a divided self stems from these conflicting cultural demands and cannot be fully explained in psychiatric terms, as it carries both moral and emancipatory dimensions. What is at stake in the anorexics' struggle is indeed the practical realization of the ideal of autonomy.[88]

If self-control is culturally defined as incompatible with the female body, then anorexia becomes a radical strategy to achieve it. Self-starving does not only aesthetically testify to the power of a will that is able to transcend the body, it also expresses an ethical standpoint that – consistently with the ideal of the autonomous man – gives absolute priority to a pure, disembodied capacity to self-govern oneself.

According to Saukko, psychiatric and public discourses are structurally unable to capture two key aspects of anorexia. First, that it contains moral and emancipatory elements – often unspoken but still held by those with the disorder.[89] Second, that these elements are celebrated in Western culture.[90] This means anorexia arises from complex social conditions as a problematic yet meaningful attempt to embody cultural ideals – ideals that, in turn, support both emancipatory and oppressive practices.[91]

Both Bordo and Saukko highlight the link between Western gender norms and the development of anorexia. For Bordo, the anorexic's alien self reflects a sublimation of the 'male' ideal of pure will. Saukko, however, sees the alien self not only as culturally shaped but also as carrying elements of moral self-determination – an expression of political resistance or social self-affirmation. Yet, despite Saukko's focus on autonomy, it remains unclear how people with anorexia can play an active role if anorexia is, in her account, largely the *result* of an unjust social structure that demands what it simultaneously renders unattainable.

A 'moral' perspective

In *Understanding Eating Disorders*, Giordano challenges the aetiology of anorexia proposed by contextual perspectives. Her critique unfolds in three main steps, calling for an approach that better captures the moral and personal dimensions at the heart of the disorder.

1. *Unverified assumption: Inappropriate expectations don't directly cause suffering.*
   What causes distress is not the expectation itself, but the individual's moral relationship to it – either through guilt (feeling personally at fault) or alienation (seeing others as blameworthy). The expectation–disappointment dynamic is morally grounded and subjectively endorsed: the person suffers because they have accepted and exercised a set of values that renders failed expectations undesirable and morally charged.
2. *Failure of the neutral approach: Contextual perspectives mirror the moral logic of anorexia.*
   By portraying anorexics as victims of harmful environments, they avoid blaming the individual but shift moral judgement onto others. This replicates the guilt-based moral framework that anorexia already relies on.[92]
3. *Logical fallacy: Correlation does not imply causation.*
   The contextual variables linked to anorexia – while helpful for understanding the experience and improving treatment – cannot be considered its cause. These factors may inform therapeutic strategies but don't explain the choices, behaviours or values of those with anorexia.[93]

Giordano argues that anorexia is not caused by familial, social or cultural contexts but emerges from the individual's moral dimension. Unlike contextual perspectives, she focuses on the person's role in shaping ethical values. In contrast, the postmodern frameworks of Saukko and Bordo portray the individual's agency as socially constructed, that is, as essentially reactive. By shifting explanation from the person to the environment, these perspectives downplay the individual's active role and overlook the moral commitments that link them to cultural ideals.

For Giordano, individuals actively interpret and respond to their culture, exercising some level of direction and control in how they engage with societal norms. The goal is not to assign blame, but to recognize the person's role in the development and persistence of anorexia and to frame it in a way that respects their identity and moral sensibility.[94] Anorexia, in this view, is a strategy to pursue self-control, purity and willpower – anchored in the belief that autonomy is morally valuable.[95] It also becomes a means of gaining power *over* the environment by leveraging the moral idea that causing suffering is wrong.

> The [anorexic] person is saying 'do you see how much you are making me suffer?' – and expects others to change accordingly. It is in fact a rather common belief that people should feel sorry for other people's suffering and do something about it. Therefore, it is common for people to try to achieve a change in others by displaying their misery to them and maybe blaming them for it (an illustrative case is that of hunger-strikers).[96]

For Giordano, morality – not the environment – is central to anorexic behaviours, values and identity. Anorexia is a coherent way of expressing deeply held moral beliefs, not merely a reaction to societal pressure. While these moral values are not reducible to mere 'reactions' to society, they are nonetheless interpretations of Western morality. In this sense, anorexia constitutes an articulation of Western culture that reveals how its moral ideals can be both empowering and weakening, liberating and oppressive. To understand anorexia fully, Giordano argues, we must consider the moral dimension of the person *and* the critique that her interpretation of social morality raises.[97]

The difference between contextual perspectives and Giordano's view is subtle but crucial. In Saukko and Bordo's accounts, anorexic beliefs are shaped by the environment. For Giordano, they emerge from the relationship between the individual and the environment. The affective dimension is phenomenologically prior both to the formation of the beliefs and to the dichotomy subject-environment.[98]

Giordano's model includes the social context only insofar as it is personally endorsed – meaning the agent is morally active in their participation in that context. While Bordo, and especially Saukko, seek to restore agency to the individual, their focus on the coercive power of culture still casts the person as reactive – either rebelling against or submitting to social norms – leaving little room for true autonomy.

Giordano, by contrast, sees no strong evidence that anorexia is caused by cultural conflict or social oppression alone. People with anorexia often articulate moral ideals in ways that reflect a personal interpretation of cultural values – one that aligns with their identity and sensibility. In this view, they are active participants in their endorsement of the cultural ideals and in the development of their 'anorexic' identity and morality. Giordano's approach thus rejects the assumption of anorexics' non-autonomy and lays the ground for an articulation of a perspective more responsive to their identity and moral perspective.

In the next chapter, I will examine current legislation on the refusal of treatment in anorexia, highlighting the legal and ethical challenges it raises. This analysis will help clarify which aspects of anorexia are recognized – or overlooked – by the law. I will build on Giordano's critique of English law, assessing whether her proposed solutions are sustainable, effective and respectful of the complexities of anorexia discussed in this chapter.

2

Anorexic Patients and Normative Gaps

The troubled relation between anorexia and law

As shown previously, people with anorexia often have conflicted and ambiguous views of their condition. Those strongly identifying with anorexia are unlikely to accept medical treatment, and those without negative attitudes towards it rarely seek help. Individuals viewing anorexia as a positive lifestyle generally do not recognize it as a disorder, especially if they see it as essential to their identity. People with anorexia usually resist changing eating behaviours or engaging in therapy due to multiple factors: fear of food, egosyntonicity with anorexia, false beliefs, low self-worth, obsessive or compulsive behaviours, high value placed on thinness and overwhelming emotional states. Refusal of life-saving interventions, like nasogastric feeding, complicates healthcare decisions, leaving professionals and families uncertain about involuntary treatment, especially when mental capacity is acknowledged by functional assessments. Typically, people with anorexia can articulate and defend their decisions and perceive forced feeding as an attack on their autonomy and as intolerable violence.

But what governs English law about the refusal of treatment of people with anorexia? There is an explicit – and ambiguous – reference to anorexia in the *Mental Capacity Act 2005: Code of Practice*:

> A person with the eating disorder anorexia nervosa may understand information about the consequences of not eating. But their compulsion not to eat might be too strong for them to ignore.[1]

Under the Mental Capacity Act 2005 (MCA)[2] a person may lack mental capacity if they cannot (1) understand, (2) remember or (3) weigh up the information needed to make a decision, or if they cannot (4) communicate her decision. None can be considered unable to decide for themselves just because their decisions are unwise or irrational.[3] Having a mental illness does not imply that the person lacks decisional capacity. The MCA explicitly states that 'a person must be assumed to have capacity unless it is established that he lacks capacity'.[4]

Competences are generally assessed by the MacCAT-T, a functional test[5] that emphasizes the cognitive and functional aspects of mental capacity.[6] Ordinarily, the MacCAT-T finds that the mental capacity of people with anorexia respects the four requirements established by the MCA.[7] However, the decisional capacity of patients with anorexia is *intuitively* considered impaired due to the eating disorder itself.

In *A Local Authority v E*, a 32-year-old intelligent woman suffering from anorexia nervosa, personality disorder, alcohol abuse and prescribed opiate dependency had been detained under the Mental Health Act 1983[8] ten times over six years. She twice requested to refuse life-saving treatment. The Court of Protection ruled that even if E was able to understand and retain the relevant information and to communicate her decisions, she could not refuse treatment since 'her obsessive fear of gaining weight made her incapable of meaningfully weighing the advantages and disadvantages of eating'.[9] As Wang points out, this case highlights the way in which the MCA is interpreted and applied: the incapacity to weigh information about food is proved by the refusal of food; that is, the diagnosis of anorexia nervosa *already* implies the incapacity to refuse naso-gastric treatment, since anorexia implies food refusal.[10] As a result, the functional test becomes redundant, the priority given to mental capacities is overridden, and the decisions regarding treatment are reduced to a decision about food. This approach conflicts with the UN Convention on the Rights of Persons with Disabilities (CRPD), which prohibits discrimination based on mental disorders. It is not inherently inappropriate to question a patient's capacity even if they meet the formal criteria set out by the MCA – indeed, there may be other conditions where such scrutiny is warranted. However, within the current legal framework, capacity must be assessed functionally and without bias towards specific diagnoses. By systematically treating anorexic patients as lacking capacity despite fulfilling the MCA criteria, current legal practices implicitly assume anorexic patients lack sufficient autonomy to make decisions like other adults with sufficient mental capacity.[11]

Even if interrelated, the problems of the current interpretation of the MCA can be divided into three groups:

1. *Reduction*: if patients with anorexia lack decisional capacity due to an inability to weigh eating consequences, refusing treatment becomes solely a food-related decision. Notably, the Royal College of Psychiatrists, Physicians, and Pathologists states that forced feeding is not merely nutritional; it involves pain, coercion and mental and physical risks.[12]
2. *Discrimination*: competence to refuse treatment is usually assessed through the functional test, yet incompetence for anorexic patients involves a different and uncommon process: a recourse to the very definition of anorexia. The conflict between the MCA and the CRPD focuses precisely on English law's prejudice regarding mental capacity of patients with anorexia.
3. *Analytical inefficiency*: using mental disorder as a 'special justification' to assess decisional incapacity prevents the functional test from capturing genuine impairments in capacity – if they exist. Thus, the current framework neglects the role and complexity of moral, emotional and affective factors.

Before discussing the current interpretation of the MCA, I would like to add two further points regarding the relation between treatment refusal and English law. The first (A) will help historically and legally to contextualize current legislation; the second (B) will focus my emphasis on the contradictions within the law.

(A) Prior to the MCA (2005), anorexic patients were usually treated under sections 2 and 3 of the Mental Health Act (MHA, 1983), though its application was problematic.[13] Section 63 states that 'the consent of a patient shall not be required for any medical treatment given to him for the mental disorder from which he is suffering'. Yet, this raises the question: Is force-feeding a treatment specifically for anorexia? The *Guidance on the Treatment of Anorexia under the Mental Health Act 1983* considers force-feeding a 'symptomatic' treatment, permissible under section 63.[14] However, this conclusion conflicts with the *Code of Practice: Mental Health Act 1983,*[15] which states that mental disorders should not automatically imply incapacity to refuse treatment. Nonetheless, refusal of force-feeding is still considered incompetent due solely to the anorexia diagnosis.

(B) The recent case of *A NHS Foundation Trust v Ms X*[16] reignited debate around interpreting the MCA concerning anorexia. Ms X suffered from severe anorexia nervosa and alcohol dependence, leading to irreversible liver disease. Although repeatedly treated under sections 2 and 3 of the MHA, forced feeding led to increased alcohol intake to cope with treatment stress. She was considered unable to decide about food but capable regarding alcohol. Her refusal of force-feeding was initially rejected, yet the NHS Trust ultimately declared:

> It was not in Ms X's best interests to be subject to further compulsory detention and treatment of her anorexia nervosa, whether under the Mental Health Act 1983 or otherwise, notwithstanding that such treatment may prolong her life. It was in her best interests, and should be declared lawful, for her treating clinicians not to provide Ms X with nutrition and hydration with which she does not comply.[17]

Even in this case the patient was found unable to decide about food due to her mental disorder, but her unaccepted decision and the judge's declaration substantially coincide: force-feeding is not an acceptable treatment. The judge and Ms X agreed that further treatment would exacerbate suffering and alcohol abuse, worsening her condition. Some might argue Ms X's decision aligned with the court's conclusion only due to peculiar (exceptional?) circumstances. However, I think that this argument cannot be defended without rejecting at all the possibility that mentally impaired persons might be autonomous in some relevant way. Ms X's and the court's decisions coincided both in outcome and rationale. Additionally, although Ms X was functionally competent, she was considered incapable because of her diagnosis. This case clearly indicates that the current application of the MCA is inadequate in its grasp of more fine-grained states of autonomy and lack of autonomy.

Food refusal, perceptual disorders and maladaptive habits

As I have outlined, the MCA recognizes the patient's decisional capacity through a functional test of mental capacity, but even when mental capacity is considered valid, their decision is not accepted due to the diagnosis of anorexia.

Criticism of this constitutes one of the main themes of Giordano's *Understanding Eating Disorder*. According to Giordano, in the majority of cases a mental illness is not explicative of certain behaviours. She admits that solid scientific data can reveal a correspondence between certain behaviour and mental impairments (e.g. the brain deterioration that causes loss of memory in Alzheimer's disease), but in most cases the diagnosis of mental disorder is 'only a short cut to describe a pattern of disturbance: it has no explanatory value'.[18] In such cases – anorexia included – the mental disorder should be understood as a description of a phenomenon disconnected from a person's autonomy. Behavioural disorder can indicate a need to investigate carefully whether the person lacks autonomy, but the behaviour itself cannot be simply considered as *caused* by the mental disorder since the definition of mental disorder coincides with the behavioural disorder.[19] As Giordano points out:

> Arguments that people diet and vomit 'because they have an eating disorder' is fallacious. Arguments that we are justified in intervening against the eating-disordered person because her behaviour is 'the result of a mental illness' are fallacious. Paternalism should not be based on such fallacious grounds.[20]

Typically, the assumption that anorexic patients lack decisional capacity arises from their difficulty weighing information about their bodies and food.[21] Other disorders that share this feature of anorexia such as the body dysmorphic disorder (characterized by the obsessive idea that parts of the body are defective) or, more emblematically, body integrity identity disorder (BIID) (a disorder in which individuals perceive one or more of their limbs as alien and request amputation), but only people with anorexia are presumed to be incompetent to decide about their body despite the results of a functional test. For example, UK law has permitted BIID patients to legally amputate limbs, and in January 2000 a surgeon at the Falkirk and District Royal Infirmary of Scotland amputated the legs of two patients with BIID.[22]

Neurological studies on the role of self-perception in anorexia indicate that there is no sufficient ground to state that the behaviour of people with anorexia is caused by perceptual disorders. Rather, studies highlight connections between emotional, affective brain regions and body image perceptions, satisfaction and size estimations.[23] Furthermore, it has been proven that people experiencing anorexia can estimate their own body as unrealistically healthy or fat, while their evaluations of others' bodies are accurate.[24] These results underline that the peculiar self-perception of people with anorexia cannot be explained by a simplistic 'perceptual disturbance' relative to, or caused by, anorexia. Rather, if the perception of body image is a process grounded in optative, emotional and affective responses[25] – as emerging evidences point out – their self-perception should be considered a consequence or a part of their moral and affective state:

> In the way they *look at* their body and *perceive* their body, people express not only what they *see*, but also how they *think* they look, how they *feel* they look, and how they *want* to look.[26]

But what about the capacity to *weigh* information about food? People with anorexia are often very well informed about food, calories and nutritional properties, but it is generally claimed that they are unable to apply this knowledge to themselves.[27] Even when people with anorexia are perfectly aware of the minimum number of calories required by the human body, they can nevertheless affirm that they need only an inadequate number of calories. It is not uncommon for people experiencing anorexia to consider themselves as an 'exception', as if the evidence valid for everyone else does not apply to them.[28]

Recent neurological studies have found abnormal dorsal striatum activity during food choice tasks in individuals with anorexia, linking this brain region to habit formation and decision-making.[29] Researchers suggest these irregularities may hinder patients' ability to adapt food choices appropriately, especially during treatments aimed at weight gain.[30] While this finding might support claims of impaired decisional capacity, such conclusions are premature. Abnormal dorsal striatum functioning is not the *cause* of their inability to use and weigh information about food, even if it is an important indicator of their difficulties in altering alimentary habits. Some people experiencing anorexia can be trapped in a catch-22 situation – and the functional test should be able to detect this – but there is no need to presuppose that this is true of *all* people with anorexia only because they have anorexia. Some people with anorexia are, in fact, able – especially if supported by family, friends and health-care professionals – to alter their eating habits and to accept the treatment.[31] Others, particularly those with severe and enduring anorexia, can be deeply aware of their incapacity to choose food and decide to refuse force-feeding. Cases such as *A NHS Foundation Trust v Ms X* show how decisions about food refusal can be substantially correct (in their best interests) even if they are not considered valid.[32]

Giordano makes an important distinction about the attitude to food: 'Instead of being used for improving health and well-being, [the information] is utilized *as a justification* for an unhealthy and clearly harmful lifestyle.'[33] But this cannot be said for every case. Refusing food cannot be reduced to a symptom of illness or neurological anomaly. As mentioned earlier, former anorexics typically view their anorexic experiences as essential to their identity. Presuming incapacity discriminates against anorexic patients, mischaracterizing deliberative 'defects' as inherently part of their identity. People with anorexia can use the information to justify a way of life that aims to fulfil certain values or moral concerns rather than to justify a harmful lifestyle; the malaise could indeed be considered a price worth paying for the achievement of what is considered high ideals.[34]

Thus, incapacity to weigh food information does not simply cause self-starvation. The refusal of food cannot merely be explained as a 'symptom' of the 'illness' or of certain anomalies of the dorsal striatum. As mentioned earlier, post-anorexics typically view their anorexic experiences as essential to their identity and self-understanding. Presuming incapacity discriminates against anorexic patients, mischaracterizing deliberative 'defects' as inherently part of their identity.

Giordano's brave claim

It's crucial to clarify that stating anorexic behaviour is not caused by a mental disorder does not imply it is always autonomous or that paternalistic intervention is never justified. Some individuals with anorexia are deeply unaware of their condition, perceiving it as normal or positive. Some cannot integrate information about food contradicting their habits or values, while others may exhibit strong ambivalence towards treatment or feel paralyzed by the fear of food. As we have seen in the section on anorexic perspectives, such cases can correspond to certain configurations of anorexia, but they do not correspond with anorexia *in toto*. Furthermore, these kinds of impairment can indeed be recognized by the functional test and do not need recourse to the definition of an eating disorder.

But what about patients with anorexia aware of their disorder who refuse treatment? Should they be free to refuse force-feeding since their capacities are considered valid by the MacCAT-T?

The main argument that sustains her solution is that anorexic behaviour is not *caused* by dysfunctions or defects in the deliberation. Rather, peculiar deliberations are an integral part of their moral and subjective standpoint. Giordano provides two additional arguments against paternalistic intervention for individuals with anorexia who maintain functional decisional capacity:

1. Intervention against a person's will is generally justified if their behaviour is non-autonomous and harmful. Even leaving aside autonomy, it remains unclear which anorexic behaviours clearly constitute harm or when the harm is sufficient to justify coercion. Repeated vomiting and severe starvation obviously endanger health. However, anorexic behaviour includes various non-harmful activities like checking weight, exercising and selecting food. Additionally, many anorexic acts pose neither immediate nor significant threats to health, making it challenging to clearly define or measure the harm involved when behaviours aren't directly life-threatening.
2. If anorexia is experienced as a means to autonomy and self-control, coercive intervention may worsen the disorder. Patients may intensify

> anorexic behaviours to regain the autonomy compromised by forced treatment. Thus, from this perspective, force-feeding can be therapeutically counterproductive.

Giordano's perspective leads her to make a (in her own terms) *brave claim*:[35]

> People with anorexia nervosa who competently decide not to be artificially fed should be respected *because* everybody is entitled to the exercise of their autonomy. … The principle of autonomy binds us to respect people's competent decisions about their life and its termination, precisely because autonomy extends also to the most difficult moments of our life.[36]

Giordano concludes that patients whose decisional capacity is validated by the MacCAT-T should be free to decide for themselves, as the law grants every competent person the freedom to self-govern. Her conclusion acknowledges the current legislation's shortcomings,[37] proposing a solution that is practical and non-discriminative towards individuals with anorexia.

The limits of value-neutral approaches

Despite Giordano's legitimate critique of English law, I believe that her *brave claim* is problematic and ultimately inadequate. In an important passage, Giordano states that there are two options for the law on treatment of patients with anorexia:

> The first option is to assess patients' competence to decide on force-feeding. This would have the advantage of guaranteeing respect for people's real competence. The downside is that lawyers and health-care professionals may risk embarking on *interminable* discussions of the nature of competence, mental illness, and autonomy of behaviour.
>
> The second option is to show that force-feeding is a treatment for the mental disorder. The advantage is a practical one. Ethical or not, the treatment for the mental disorder is enforceable by law. Thus, the patient's life is saved and health-care professionals are protected. The downside here is the difficulty to show that food is a psychiatric therapy.[38]

Criticizing the second option, she constructs a third way out, the *brave claim*. However, she dedicates less analysis to the first option, dismissing it due to potential 'interminable' discussions. She observes:

> The fact that a person has received a diagnosis of mental illness does not give us reason to assume that she is incompetent. It may instead give us reason to investigate further her capacity to consent … However, this position is hard to defend … Saying that we should assess the capacity of eating-disordered people to refuse treatment gives rise to a number of difficult questions, and may give rise to an *interminable* debate on the nature of competence. What does it mean to be competent to refuse treatment? The law has provided an answer, but one that is open to discussion and that may sometimes raise more problems than it resolves.[39]

Giordano accurately points out that healthcare and legal professionals cannot resolve philosophical debates about capacity and autonomy when deciding treatment. To overcome this obstacle, she proposes a practical solution aligning with current legislation's limits while challenging its flaws: individuals considered competent via the functional test should have the right to refuse treatment.[40] However, while rightly contesting the law's approach, she neglects to challenge its underlying value-neutral stance. Specifically, she overlooks two important points: a purely functional test might fail to capture nuanced autonomy states, and it could be essential to consider reasons and values when assessing autonomy. Anorexia may thus highlight not only the limitations of the MCA's procedural method but also the wider value-neutral framework in which it is embedded.

Why does Giordano ignore this possibility? Possibly due to her commitment to a procedural conception of autonomy. She argue that the procedural conception of autonomy – an action is autonomous if the process of deliberation is correct – 'guarantees respect both for a person's welfare and for the way in which she wishes to shape her life autonomously',[41] whereas the substantive one – an action is autonomous on the base of the rationality of its outcome – 'leads to the justification of an authoritarian attitude towards the patient and disregard for patient autonomy'.[42] According to Giordano, health-care professionals may legitimately prevent the harmful conduct of a person if they lack autonomy regarding that particular action or choice, but the assessment of autonomy should focus only on thought processes, not content.

According to Giordano, autonomy cannot be assessed taking into account values and reasons because this approach implies the introduction of a pattern of 'good' reasons and values that have to be fulfilled in order to be considered autonomous. In her view, the substantive approach leads to an authoritarian approach to reasons and values, and for this reason it cannot be endorsed without disregarding patients' autonomy. But is this really the case?

Recently, scholars have argued that excluding values and reasons from autonomy assessments underestimates their significance. In this regard, Diana Meyers raises a crucial point. She affirms that any conception of autonomy, *including value-neutral conceptions*, has some values 'explicitly or implicitly invoked to explicate the reflective procedure or motivational structure that renders choices and actions autonomous'.[43] In order to obtain a more fine-grained image of the different ways in which values can be included or excluded in a theory of autonomy, Meyers distinguishes two axes. Along the first axis – the *Directivity Axis* – the account of autonomy is framed by different degrees of prescribed values, ranging from value-neutral theories (no prescription of values) to value-saturated theories (prescription of certain values), with various degrees of value-laden conception (limitation of certain oppressive conditions) in the middle; along the second axis – the *Constitutivity Axis* – the account of autonomy is framed by a pattern of qualitatively distinct sets of values that establish the particular notion of autonomy in question (what Meyers calls '*constitutive value sets*' of a theory[44]). Following Meyers's analysis of autonomy theories, Giordano's dichotomy between procedural and substantive conceptions of autonomy appears misleading: 'Even rational choice theory – a paradigm of value neutrality – rests on a constitutive set of epistemic values including consistency, transitivity, and knowledge of pertinent facts.'[45]

Although Meyers maintains a value-neutral stance on decisional capacity, she argues a coherent autonomy theory must recognize its position on the Constitutivity Axis – acknowledging the function and conditions underlying its inherent values. Discussion of the relation between values and autonomy is not only *interminable*, as Giordano claims, but also *perfectible*. Any theory of autonomy always and unavoidably assumes certain values that – if articulated – are open to discussion and revision, but they are notwithstanding operative, even in the current legal approach. Meyers – following Andrea Westlund[46] – argues that, for instance, the moral values of interpersonal answerability 'do not predict what autonomous people will choose to do or become other than being autonomous'.[47]

Along the Directivity Axis, as we have seen, there is a graduated scale of positions ranging from value-neutral (no prescription of values) to value-saturated (prescription of certain values). Meyers affirms that there are various degrees of value-laden positions (limitation of the agent's conditions of oppression) in the middle, but, whereas the value-saturated position has various degrees in itself (depending on the rigidity and the demands of the prescriptions), the value-neutral position is a sort of 'level zero' or asymptote. In fact, following Meyers's argument, even the most value-neutral theories are sustained by – and sustain – certain values and reasons. A coherent value-neutral theory of autonomy – a theory that reflects on its own moral commitments, such as Meyers's – would be arranged on the value-laden side of the Directivity Axis because it would – in some way – consider values and reasons in the assessment of autonomy, and so it would no longer be value-neutral. Meyers, instead, stresses the idea that a coherent value-utilizing theory can still be value-neutral: value-neutral theories consider that it is possible autonomously to conform to oppressive norms, while value-laden theories do not. I think that this kind of distinction tends to generate incomprehension since the important data – at least from a bioethical point of view – is that *value-utilizing theories of autonomy recognize the role of values and reasons in the assessment of decisional capacity*. Given the pervasiveness of values in any theory of autonomy, the label 'value-neutral' itself is misleading. My proposal is to reconfigure the Directivity Axis with value-saturated (prescription of values), *intermediary* value-laden (prescription of social condition) and *dialogical* value-laden positions (prescription of condition of existence of values).

In order to assess autonomy taking into account reasons and values, it is not necessary to judge the content or the outcome of their choices and actions and to ascribe certain values to them; not to presuppose that certain social conditions necessarily impair autonomy. Instead, it requires recognizing that reasons and values exist under certain conditions, and these conditions significantly influence autonomy. From this perspective, the MCA exhibits critical inadequacies concerning autonomy's moral and rational foundations.

Giordano's *brave claim* cannot resolve the dilemma of the refusal of force-feeding because it disregards the problems highlighted by law: the functional test is inadequate, and reasons and values are pivotal features not only of autonomy but also of any theoretical approach to autonomy. Giordano's recourse to the *brave claim* is drastic and potentially harmful, especially if considered that scholars have developed – especially in the last two decades – broader and more fine-grained accounts of autonomy and human agency that could enable lawyers and health-care professionals to gain a deeper insight into decisional capacity without producing any undesirable impasse.

The shortcomings evident in both the current application of the MCA and Giordano's *brave claim* reveal deeper issues stemming from a reductive, value-neutral view of human agency.[48] In the following chapter, I extend my critique of value-neutral and procedural approaches to autonomy, highlighting their structural defects while acknowledging their merits. This critical task will introduce the first relational conditions required for autonomy and will help show how the failure to recognize adequately the claims made by people with anorexia is connected to an unsustainable epistemological background that denies the possibility of acknowledging others' reasons. Specifically, employing Taylor's critique of monologicity, I will illustrate how the current epistemological framework rests on a flattened view of human agents, unable to grasp their most fine-grained claims, such as those made by people with anorexia.

3

The Separation between Autonomy and Reasons

As we have seen, English law establishes no correlation between mental capacity and decision content. Lord Donaldson, in the case Re. Miss T, stated clearly that '[a competent adult's] right of choice … exists notwithstanding that the reasons for making the choice are rational, irrational, unknown or even non-existent'.[1] If we rely only on the functional test to assess the capacity of patients with anorexia,[2] then they must be deemed capable of refusing treatment – regardless of whether their decision is based on rational reasons, irrational motives or no identifiable reason at all. In the previous chapter, I critiqued both English law's official approach and Giordano's alternative, highlighting their flawed understanding of reasons and values in autonomy. Following Meyers, I argued that every theory of autonomy inevitably incorporates certain reasons and values and that a coherent theory must acknowledge this.

My aim in this chapter is to articulate the reasons sustaining the separation between reasons and autonomy assumed both in the MCA and in Giordano's view. I will outline two influential conceptions – internalism and externalism – demonstrating that externalism is incompatible with liberal frameworks, as it assumes paternalistic interventions when patients refuse actions justified by external reasons. However, even internalism cannot adequately address the relevant issues about reasoning and values, failing to protect patients with anorexia due to its oversimplified conception of human agency. Ultimately, I argue that autonomy should be conceptualized differently to overcome this internalist-externalist impasse. Importantly, in this chapter I will make extensive use of the language and terminology adopted by defenders of liberalism (in particular in reference to terms such as 'motivational set', 'motivation' and 'motives'). This choice must not be intended as an acceptance of the liberal framework, but rather as a direct consequence of my aim to criticize liberalism 'from within' and 'immanently', that is, by assuming what is acceptable to liberalism in order to bring this philosophical framework to its inherent limits and to make clear its peculiar contradictions. This is strategic for my argument as both the MCA and the internalist perspective are grounded in a liberal framework.

Why internalism?

Internalism refers to explaining phenomena like meaning, truth, motivation and reasons in relation to internal factors. Here, I use internalism specifically regarding *reasons*. In his famous article 'Internal and External Reasons',[3] Bernard Williams defines the internalist conception of reasons as a way of interpreting propositions of the form: 'A has reasons to φ'; thus 'A has some motive which will be served or furthered by his φing'.[4] To have a reason for an action, from an internalist point of view, is to have a subjective motivational set that can be served by that action. Actions are, in this sense, *explained* by reasons, and reasons are in turn grounded in subjective motives. Williams illustrates internalism with someone desiring gin in a bottle, unaware that it contains petrol. Williams explains that this shows that it is incorrect to say that 'B has a reason to drink the content of the bottle', because if B knew that the content of the bottle was petrol and not gin, they (presumably) would not have had any motive to drink it. They want gin, not petrol. Thus, according to Williams, a correct understanding of the relevant information about possible actions and decisions is a necessary condition of having a reason. Even if B is motivated to drink gin, he has no genuine reason to drink the contents of the bottle.[5] B could have a reason to drink the petrol if he were motivated to commit suicide, for example. And Hume has a reason to prefer the destruction of the whole world to the scratching of his finger, insofar as he wishes for that to take place.[6] 'Internal reasons' are not understood in terms of rational conditions, but in terms of desires: on this view (as I attack the view, rather than endorsing it!), 'morality is not a matter of reason, but of contingent wants'.[7]

Clearly, then, one of the ethical and political implications of the internalist conception of reasons is the establishment of moral subjectivism.[8] For if the ultimate ground of reasons is the motivational set of the agent, there are no reasons independent of what the agent happens to want. In this view, moral rules and imperatives apply only to those agents who are already motivated to join the moral domain in which those rules and imperatives are valid: agents who *want* to do so. For example, a card sharper cannot have a reason against defrauding others if honesty is not within their motivational set. From an internalist point of view, there is no correlation between responsiveness to moral demands and reasons:[9] the card sharper is not irrational in his defrauding (or, he has reason to defraud people) because he does not care about the whole moral dimension in which not defrauding is understood as important. The internalist account regards agents' motives as *final*, one might say.[10] Internalism sees moral reasoning as dependent entirely on personal motivations; thus, moral obligations hold significance only within shared moral commitments.

The connection between the internalist understanding of reasons and the MCA – and liberal[11] legislation more generally – is explicit.[12] Liberal accounts of autonomy, as endorsed by the MCA, stress the normative neutrality of the concept, stating that only those reasons that the person accepts – even if irrational or inconsistent[13] – can be taken into account in assessing mental capacity. Giordano's *brave claim* aligns similarly. From an internalist perspective, reasons may appear unintelligible because they arise from internal, often concealed motivations. Reasons depend exclusively on personal beliefs, interests and desires, which remain immune to broader moral evaluations. De facto, the primacy of the motivational set of the agent renders inquiry into reasons in relation to mental capacity impossible or, in the best case, accessory.

However, the internalist perspective has the – apparent – advantage of guaranteeing a value-neutral and non-discriminative approach to autonomy. This is why internalism is so closely compatible with liberal legislation and appealing in relation to questions of multiculturalism, pluralism and ethical disagreement: reasons are all equal because they are all valid, just inasmuch as they happen to be grounded in individuals' motivational sets. From an internalist point of view, it is not only legitimate, but also *more prudent*, not to consider reasons at all, given that their understanding is ultimately grounded on a particular – and therefore potentially discriminatory – shared moral commitment. In short, internalism is the formal conclusion of Hume's sophisticated subjectivism.

However, as previously discussed, applying internalism creates substantial contradictions, especially regarding anorexia and medical decisions. Patients with anorexia often refuse treatment due to complex motivations, such as egosyntonic symptoms, false beliefs, deep identification with anorexia, feelings of unworthiness or overwhelming anxieties. In all these cases, the reasoning of patients with anorexia is consistent with the MCA's conception of mental capacity: they are indeed able to understand and 'weigh'[14] the relevant information connected to medical decisions. As noted in Chapter 2, this conclusion is deeply problematic because: (1) it conflates medical decisions regarding food with a decision regarding *solely* food; (2) it discriminates against anorexic patients despite positive capacity assessments; and (3) it fails to justify paternalistic interventions consistent with liberal principles of equality and personal freedom.[15] The MCA's abstract and amoral stance disregards critical factors like values, identity and moral reasoning, inadequately addressing mental capacity impairments without unfairly linking anorexia to incapacity. In order to overcome these problems, internalism's opposite, *externalism*, is often brought into play.

Why (not) externalism?

According to Williams, the externalist conception of reasons reads propositions structured in the form of 'A has reasons to φ' as *not* implying that 'A has some motive which will be served or furthered by his φing'.[16] Thus, from an externalist perspective, reasons for actions are not dependent on personal motivations but reflect objective truths or facts. The attractiveness of externalism relies on the idea that reasons are reflective of objective truths or statements of facts, so that it is possible to assess the legitimacy of actions, beliefs and motives on the grounds of this correspondence. In this account, an agent 'has a reason' when they are acting in the light of a *correct* understanding of the context.

Williams critiques externalism, arguing it fails to explain actions convincingly. Agents, Williams claims, act for reasons, and their reasons must therefore be able to explain their actions. But external reasons are supposed to explain an action in the light of something that is not 'within' the agent (i.e. in the agent's motivational set). So how can they explain an agent's action? A's decision (let's say) to share his food with B cannot be explained by the fact that B is starving. That 'B is starving' is an objective state of things external to the agent, and, as such, it cannot *cause* A's action or *motivate* him to act in a certain way. Williams introduces an example:

> Owen's family urge on him the necessity and importance of his joining the army, since all his male ancestors were soldiers, and family pride requires him to do the same. Owen Wingrave has no motivation to join the army at all, and all his desires lead in another direction: he hates everything about military life and what it means. His family might have expressed themselves by saying that *there was a reason for Owen to join the army.*[17]

The central feature of external reasons is that they can be true independently of the agent's motivational set. But if we hold with Williams that 'nothing can explain an agent's (intentional) actions except something that motivates him so to act',[18] external reasons are not able to explain actions since they lack any psychological connection to the agent that would render an action intelligible. Owen's family's external reason would not explain Owen's actions even if he did join the army because it would not be *Owen's* reason. There is no connection to his motivational set. Williams argues that if Owen joins the army, it is because he 'now believes that it is a reason *for him* to do so that his family has a tradition of military honour',[19] or, in other words, Owen joins the army because he has an internal reason to join the army.[20] There is now, in Williams' terms, a connection between the reason and the agent.

Especially if described in a general form[21] – as I have done – the externalist conception of reasons not only appears implausible since it cannot explain action; it is also problematic from an ethical and political point of view, particularly if considered from a liberal stance.[22] For if reasons can be independent of the motivational set of the agent, the normative power of reasons shifts from the individual to some external domain that it is not under his or her direct control. For instance, a society might enforce compulsory exercise, citing health benefits.[23] On this view, moral rules and moral imperatives apply indiscriminately to all agents, independently of the fact that they are not motivated to subscribe to the moral framework in which those rules and imperatives hold sway.

From an externalist point of view, then, the normative power of an external reason (e.g. it is wrong to defraud) is not invalidated by the absence in the card sharper of some motivational set regarding the importance of not defrauding. On the contrary, the fraudulent actions of the card sharper are irrational because they are not responsive to the moral background in which not defrauding is important. But then *where* is the reason for the card sharper to desist, or for Owen to join the army? Do these reasons really *exist*?

Liberal thinkers, including Giordano, find externalism unattractive precisely because it conflicts with liberal values of autonomy and normative neutrality. An agent could be indifferent to the benefits offered by physical activity and have a reason to refuse compulsory exercise because, for them (let's say), it is important to have a lazy lifestyle and spend their time accordingly. Even if external reasons can be disconnected from moral backgrounds (mathematical reasons, for example), participation in a domain external to the motivations of the individual remains a necessary condition of rational agency. As a consequence, externalism reconfigures the conditions of exercising autonomy in light of the normative primacy of objective reasons at the expense of agents' *desires*.

In the liberal tradition, autonomy is understood as the capacity of the agent to follow *their own* reasons, *their own* beliefs.[24] But if reasons for action are external, it is presumably right to follow them even in those cases in which the agent is not even *able* to recognize their normative authority. The liberal problem with externalism is that, insofar as it is applied in practice, it presupposes a strong form of paternalism. In conclusion, externalism cannot fulfil the liberal ideal of a self-*determining* individual. If Owen joins the army without wanting to, external obligations, not personal choices, would govern his life.

Internalism and egosyntonicity

At first glance, internalism appears intuitive and straightforward. It seems natural that actions cannot be autonomous unless the agent has a motive to perform them. However, I suspect this apparent clarity stems largely from cultural assumptions that internalism is inherently correct. Let's look at my previous pseudo-rhetorical question: *how can an action be autonomously performed if the agent does not have a motive to perform that action*? Although seemingly reasonable, this question contains two problematic assumptions. First, it *presupposes* that autonomous actions always require a motive.[25] Second, it assumes an autonomous agent must possess identifiable mental content – motives, beliefs and desires – corresponding to reasons. But are these assumptions necessarily true? Do reasons genuinely reside within individuals' minds?

In assuming that actions 'start from the inside', internalism assumes an internal domain in which the individual is free to develop and manage the source of her intentional actions. The 'internalist' agent is a sort of *black box* with an input – the information – and an output – the decision. Inside the black box, the information is processed in the light (in the shadow?) of the personal motives and beliefs of the agent. Provided the individual's cognitive processes – the box's 'structure' – are intact, their decisions are considered rational, regardless of their specific content. Under this model, others can evaluate only whether an individual processes information correctly and communicates decisions effectively, not their internal motivations. The individual alone administers this internal domain, defining their reasons by acting in alignment with them. However, I contend this perspective is flawed and inadequate. First, it creates significant practical issues, especially in medical and legal contexts; second, it fails to differentiate clearly between rational and irrational decisions.

To illustrate these issues, consider internalism's application to clinical cases, specifically patients with anorexia who are reluctant to accept treatment. As discussed in Chapter 1, one of the most severe, intrusive and blurred aspects of anorexia is how closely its symptoms align with the patient's own beliefs and values – known as egosyntonic beliefs.[26] Many anorexic patients struggle to maintain a non-anorexic identity, experiencing difficulty in abandoning what they perceive as their 'real' self. Often, their motivational set aligns with anorexia's symptoms, especially during the disorder's early stages, leading them to see their actions as entirely consistent with their genuine beliefs. Furthermore, anorexic patients may not view their condition as a disorder but instead regard it as a positive, reflectively endorsed lifestyle. As Chapter 1 indicated, only patients capable of seeing anorexia as distinct and conflicting with their authentic self could reasonably be considered in a 'transitional stage' towards recovery.[27] Most others, particularly those early in the disorder and without support, find it difficult to distinguish their identity from anorexia or develop a negative view of the disorder *in solitude* – usually requiring support from others (family, friends and health carers) to recognize anorexia as a harmful condition.

How, then, does internalism address individuals with egosyntonic symptoms? Given that anorexic individuals usually pass functional assessments – demonstrating their ability to understand, retain and weigh information and communicate decisions – and their actions align with their motivational sets, internalism must conclude that these outcomes are rational. This is precisely the stance Giordano adopts, arguing that anorexic patients passing the functional test should have the freedom to refuse treatment.

But as I argued earlier, such a conclusion is deeply problematic and ultimately unsustainable. Psychiatrists, post-anorexics and some patients with anorexia agree that anorexia interferes with personal identity and with the moral and motivational set of the agent in a manner that cannot be detected by the functional test.[28] In the words of Participant 36:

> [Anorexia] feels like there's two of you inside, like there's another half of you, which is my anorexia and then there's the real [Self], the real me, the logic part of me and it's a constant battle between the two … The real me is what I use to fight against it and to motivate me to want to beat it and get well. I truly believe that, that if there wasn't any me left, if there was none of me inside of me then I would have let it kill me by now. [The idea of the real me] is very helpful. If I didn't have that, then – I mean, I know people who haven't got that, and they're very much stuck in their recovery, perhaps

> won't ever recover, yet I know people who have recovered who, like me, very, know the difference between the two.[29]

I do not want here to investigate the philosophical and psychological questions underlying the issue of the unity or multiplicity of the self. Rather, my focus is on a recurrent way in which decisional capacity in anorexic patients is framed. Considering insights from people with anorexia and post-anorexics, anorexia emerges as a mode of self-control that can – at least temporarily – spiral out of control. People with anorexia and post-anorexics agree that egosyntonic symptoms can become overwhelming, disrupting rationality. Some describe anorexia as involving two conflicting selves – the 'anorexic self' and the 'true self' – while others perceive anorexia as inseparable from their identity, struggling nonetheless to distance themselves from the disorder. Even when psychological functions are intact, such actions cannot be considered fully rational or authentic. Without adequate support, anorexic individuals be at the mercy of their own motives and beliefs and lose the capacity to reflect autonomously – an issue undetectable by functional assessments alone. The core problem in assessing mental capacity in anorexia involves more than just cognitive functioning; it centers on how individuals manage – or fail to manage – their identity, morality, beliefs and motivations. If this is the case – and many psychiatrists, post-anorexics and people with anorexia in treatment think it is[30] – internalism fails structurally to acknowledge these nuanced difficulties that render certain decisions at least partly irrational. In my view, this issue isn't just an exception or a minor flaw in internalism, but evidence that the theory does not fit humans and that another way to look at ourselves and to autonomy is needed.

Internalism, Delusional Beliefs, Lack of Self-Esteem and Self-Worth

Motives are understood by internalism as internal forces driving the actions that constitute the originality and identity of the agent: their content is 'private' and accessible only to their 'owner', in first person. Only the individual can authentically recognize their motives; others can assess procedural psychological functions but not the genuine content of motives. How is it possible to know that an agent is acting under the influence of delusional beliefs? How can autonomy be assessed if an individual lacks motivation to reflect on their actions and decisions? In his *Free Agent and Self-Worth*, Paul Benson offers this example:

> Imagine a [woman that falls into] helplessness and disorientation as a result of a profound change in her view of herself. … The husband [has] his wife's interests in mind. The trouble is that he is a physician, and although he has kept up with the best medical science of his day (the latter decades of the nineteenth century), that science does not understand women's health very well. He regards women who are excitable, who have active imaginations and strong passions, and who are prone to emotional outbursts in public as suffering from a serious psychological illness … The protagonist has the suspect traits, her husband makes the standard diagnosis, and the 'hysterical wife' ends up isolated, feeling rather crazy. … The woman [does not] resist the process by which her beliefs and desires were altered in the wake of her diagnosis, if she were to attend reflectively to that process. For she arrives at her sense of incompetence and estrangement from her conduct on the basis of reasons that are accepted by a scientific establishment which is socially validated and which she trusts.[31]

Benson introduces an example of *gaslighting*,[32] a form of psychological abuse in which a person induces cognitive dissonance, low self-esteem and psychological dependency in the victim by weakening their confidence in their own mental capacity.[33] Notably, from an internalist perspective, there is nothing inherently wrong with the woman's beliefs and motives in Benson's case. Each person is entitled to act according to their motivational set, and 'good' or 'right' reasons are solely those recognized by the individual.

But what happens when, as in Benson's example, the agent is immersed in a context that provides only autonomy-devaluing beliefs and motives?[34] Internalism links reasoning capacity to the agent's accurate understanding of information but ignores the influence of relational and cultural contexts on motive and belief formation. As Benson illustrates, the agent's ability to evaluate the validity of her motives depends not just on psychological or neurological functioning but on her relational environment. The woman, embedded in a context that views her as incapable, internalizes this judgement. She begins to mistrust her beliefs and question her motivations.

An internalist might object that it is not legitimate to conclude that the woman's motivational set is incompatible with her autonomy, given that only she can understand her motives – she can, after all, choose to live in a subordinate manner for some 'private' reason.[35] But what kind of knowledge is a knowledge that can be obtained only by one agent in the world? What, furthermore, would a *misunderstanding* in relation to this knowledge look like? And how could a mistake be recognized by the only agent in possession of that knowledge? These questions point to a basic and deep-rooted assumption of internalism: *the idea of a direct, unmediated, and infallible access to motives and the possibility of private knowledge.*[36]

This is a critical point. Internalism assumes that informed, cognitively functional agents cannot misinterpret their motives. But this is clearly false, as demonstrated by Benson's example and by people with anorexia experiencing egosyntonic symptoms. If agents are thought to have direct, privileged access to their motives, then misunderstandings – precisely like those seen in anorexia – become inexplicable. If only the agent can be in an epistemic position to understand their motives, then those whose understanding is flawed are left without recourse. Yet this, too, is false. The process of recognizing one's motives is not just internal but takes place in a dialogical process. Agents develop and revise motives, reasons and beliefs in conversation with or in opposition to 'significant' others.[37]

> We don't just learn the languages in dialogue and then go on to use them for *our own purposes.* We are of course expected to develop our opinions, outlook, stances towards things, and to a considerable degree through solitary reflection. But this is not how things work with important issue, like the definition of our identity. We define our identity always in dialogue with, sometimes in struggle against, the things our significant others want to see in us. Even after we outgrow some of these others – our parents, for instance – and they disappear from our lives, the conversation with them continues within us as long as we live.[38]

Personal reasons are accessible to others insofar as they are constituted in relation to, or against, the relational context in which the agent is embedded. Furthermore, certain values, such as self-worth and self-esteem, are inseparable from the capacity to develop and apply a motivational set.

By treating an agent's motivational set as *private property*, internalism overlooks the essential connection between motives and relational context. This blind spot prevents recognition of dysfunctions in decisional capacity linked either to the content of motivational sets or to the social environments in which agents are embedded. These problems – both theoretical and practical – cannot be solved by or within internalism.

Externalism, Irrationality, Paternalism

As previously discussed, externalism severs the connection between reasons and the agent's motivational set. Under this view, actions are not expressions of internal motivation but reflections of one's capacity – or incapacity – to identify and follow reasons. Moral imperatives apply universally, regardless of an agent's personal disposition or willingness to act on them. Specifically, an agent acts autonomously only 'if and only if she is able to form her actions on the basis of her values *and* she is able to form her values on the basis of what is True and Good'.[39]

For externalists, self-governance means aligning actions with the objective reasons embedded in each context. If someone faints in the street (absent any extraordinary circumstances), there is, from an externalist view, a reason for anyone present to help. The motivation behind helping is irrelevant; the essential point is whether the person is *responsive* to the reason – 'human life is important'. Someone might not think that 'human life is important' is a reason for action, but for externalism this would constitute a proof of the agent's incapacity to be responsive to that reason and, therefore, of their capacity to act rationally and autonomously in that context.

What does this imply for anorexic reasoning? Assuming mental disorders impair mental functions and can be treated, externalism holds that there is always a reason to treat those affected – regardless of their personal beliefs about treatment. Whether a person with anorexia believes treatment is beneficial or not is irrelevant. From this view, any reasoning that deviates from objective, external reasons – such as the imperative to protect life and health – is invalid. Thus, when patients with anorexia refuse treatment, externalism sees their reasoning as irrational and therefore not admissible in medical decision-making.

From this, it is clear that externalism's conclusion about people with anorexia reasoning is problematic on many levels. In such cases, refusal of treatment may be a valid and rational option, particularly given the invasiveness and distress caused by forced feeding.

1. The justification for treating someone with a mental disorder also depends on the likelihood of therapeutic success. Current treatments for anorexia fail in approximately 20 per cent of cases. Some patients – like Ms E – have undergone treatment for over a decade without success. Psychiatrists note that treatment is far less effective for patients who do not develop a non-anorexic identity early on.[40] For these patients, given the failure of the medical procedure applied, refusal of treatment can be reasonably considered a valid option for the patient from an *objective* point of view. Indeed, with forced-feeding being a very invasive treatment, it constitutes a source of great suffering for the patient.
2. Many psychiatrists argue that coercive treatment can worsen patients' struggles with self-control and self-worth. Viewing refusal – especially early in the disorder – as either unquestionably valid or plainly irrational is therapeutically risky. As we saw in the first chapter, anorexic reasoning is a complex, variable and sometimes ambiguous phenomenon, and it is reductive to consider it as just irrational, as simply one particular instance of an agent's inability to recognize a reason as such.
3. Many psychiatrists think that coercive approaches to anorexia can worsen the already problematic issues that patients with anorexia have with self-control and self-worth. While considering patients' refusal (especially in the early stages of the disorder) as straightforward is equally problematic, looking at their decisions and reasoning as simply irrational is dangerous from a therapeutic point of view. As we saw in the first chapter, there is no single and stable manner in which patients consider anorexia.

4. Many people with anorexia and post-anorexic patients consider anorexia a beneficial lifestyle. While in some cases (generally for post-anorexic patients) the integration of anorexic reasoning in the life of the patient permits a 'good' life (both according to the patients and to their friends and families) in other cases anorexic reasoning is integrated in a self-destructive and overwhelming manner (even if, especially in the early stages of the disorder, the patient may not accept such a description). There is no clear line distinguishing 'positive' from 'negative' integration, nor are there clear criteria for determining when anorexic behaviours amount to sufficient harm to justify coercion. Moreover, anorexic behaviour is not always reducible to self-harm, as it includes a broad range of non-harming acts such as weight checking, exercise and food selection. To assume that anorexic reasoning is necessarily irrational is highly problematic.
5. Externalism holds that correct decisions align with reasons that exist independently of an individual's motivational set. From a liberal perspective,[41] this constitutes a strong form of paternalism, as it limits individual liberty without considering the agent's will. The values prescribed by externalism – and the coercive potential of its paternalism – stand in conflict with core liberal ideals of autonomy and non-interference.

The issues outlined underscore the limitations of externalism in accounting for anorexic reasoning. Both individuals with anorexia and post-anorexic patients emphasize that anorexia touches on dimensions far beyond its psychiatric definition – dimensions essential to their moral self-understanding and identity. These aspects of morality and identity lie outside the narrow set of 'good' reasons recognized by externalism.

Reasons are not simply internal or external; they are neither 'in the mind' nor 'out in the world' in the way a table exists in space or a visual field exists in perception. As Wittgenstein and Taylor argue, human agents are *constitutively* embedded in a *space of reasons*. Reasons are not a *private property* of the individual or an *aspect* of the world; reasons constitute the domain in which human agents act.

In the next section, I shall develop this suggestion by thinking further about the internalist account of reasons.

Monological autonomy

While both the MCA and Giordano rely on an internalist conception of reasons, internalism – as we've seen – fails to deliver the benefits promised by its value-neutral stance. So how else might we approach the problem? In Chapter 2, I drew on Meyers's double-axis theory to critique Giordano's *brave claim*. Meyers argues that every theory is normative, whether implicitly or explicitly. Value-neutral accounts, by denying this, become inherently misleading. Let's examine this more closely.

How might internalism appear when viewed through Meyers's framework? Internalism claims not to rely on any constitutive set of values. It treats the capacity to form and apply a motivational set as morally neutral – morality, in this view, is a product of the agent's motivational set, not a precondition. But what, then, is the moral backdrop of internalism? What values does it actually presuppose? I want to explore the idea that by identifying internalism's normative underpinnings, we might better understand its contradictions – and possibly avoid them.

The central question is this: what kind of conception of autonomy does internalism implicitly assume? Internalism is grounded in a view of autonomy that places strong emphasis on the agent's *epistemological independence*. It frames the moral and rational life of human agents as essentially disengaged – from the world, and from others. More specifically, it treats agents' reasoning capacities as autonomous from social normativity and disconnected from the relational dynamics that make others' claims meaningful.[42]

This framework divides the world and the agent into two separate causal domains: the *public* domain of facts and the *private* domain of self-generated norms. From an internalist standpoint, protecting autonomy means defending this private sphere and shielding the agent's rational independence from external influence.[43] In this conception, to be autonomous is not only to act in light of one's own reasons but also to constitute *their own* reasons and values in the private and independent domain of their mind.

Let me develop these initial thoughts by following Taylor's formulation of autonomy as connected to internalism by calling it *monological.*[44] According to Taylor, there are three fundamental notions correlated to a monological conception of autonomy:[45]

1. Subjects are ideally detached.
2. Reason is fundamentally instrumental.
3. Society is essentially atomistic.

The first idea concerns the autonomy of the subject: agents are autonomous insofar as they are able to see and understand themselves as independent of others and the world. The second, stemming from the first, concerns the nature of autonomous reasoning. Because the agent is detached, their relation to the world and others is *instrumental.* This does not mean that the agent necessarily relates to others in an egoistic way, but rather that their connection to others is always indirect, in contrast to the *direct* relationship the agent has with themselves. The agent's actions are responses to their motivational set, so any engagement with others is ultimately filtered through self-interest. The third idea extends this model into the social context. A society made up of detached subjects, each acting through instrumental reasoning, can only be understood as a heterogeneous set of individuals pursuing their own individual goals.[46]

Together, these three notions characterize the monological conception of autonomy at the heart of the constitutive value set of internalism. Despite its claims to neutrality and universality, internalism is deeply committed to promoting autonomy and freedom. As Taylor emphasizes, this commitment is inseparable from a *moral* interest in discovering and expressing one's authentic self. Internalism, even if implicitly, is invested in this project. But as we've seen, its strategy is flawed. The internalist model treats epistemological independence as both a necessary and sufficient condition for identity formation. Yet the case of patients with anorexia shows that this is not always true. First, in some key situations, it is not possible to understand and articulate one's own identity and reasons without the help of others;[47] and second, the development of the capacity to understand and articulate the self, as well as the capacity to acknowledge and follow reasons, is, as Taylor claims, dialogically constituted:

> We become full human agents, capable of understanding ourselves, and hence of defining an identity, through our acquisition of a rich human language of expression … But we are inducted into language in exchange with others. No one acquires the languages needed for self-definition on their own. We are introduced to them through exchanges with others who matter to us … The genesis of the human mind is in this sense not 'monological', not something each accomplishes on his or her own, but dialogically. Moreover, this is not just a fact about *genesis,* which can be ignored later on. It's not just that we learn the languages in dialogue and then can go on to use them for our own purposes on our own … We define [our identity] always in dialogue with, sometimes in struggle against, the identities our significant others want to recognise in us.[48]

Furthermore, the idea of private reasons and motives is no more plausible than its externalist counterpart. As I've argued, how can we speak of error if it's only recognizable by one person? Is it possible to speak of errors in such cases? It seems not. But then, how could we speak of reasons at all, in the absence of the possibility of error? If it is not possible to understand what is excluded by the reasons (i.e. error) it becomes impossible to understand the reason too, and a reason that cannot be understood cannot be a reason.

As Wittgenstein reminds us, *contradiction is to be regarded, not as a catastrophe, but as a wall indicating that we can't go on here*. It is possible to go beyond the impasse generated by internalism, but it is also necessary to understand *where* we cannot go and *why* we desire to go where we cannot go.[49] Internalism, as a monological conception of autonomy and of the agent, aims to guarantee autonomy through a value-neutral and functional account of the agent. It offers two promises: (1) a neutral approach to values and reasons, and (2) assurance that the individual can self-govern.

The issue isn't just that these promises go unfulfilled – it's that they're ultimately unsustainable. Meyers's idea of constitutive value sets makes clear that no theoretical or personal perspective is entirely detached: any perspective presupposes the presence of a background in which certain elements are understood as relevant and others not. And proper psychological or neurological functioning alone does not ensure autonomy. Autonomy is not only about inference-making or memory; it is also deeply tied to how agents are situated within the dialogical contexts in which they act.

As Paul Benson puts it, an autonomous agent is able not only to express their interests and motives in their actions, but also to regard 'herself as being in an appropriate position to speak for her decision and actions in response to potential criticisms, irrespective of whether her actions actually issue from her deepest or reflectively acceptable motives or values'.[50] Similarly, Andrea Westlund holds that autonomy depends on the relational capacity to consider oneself answerable to critics regarding one's reasons for actions.[51] These relational conditions do not imply fixed moral or rational commitments (they are not externalist), but they permit the agent to act in a way that secures both their dialogical accountability and their status as a moral and a political agent.[52] In short, such values do not predict what the agent will choose or how they will act, but they allow the agent to exercise autonomy in the relational context – the context in which autonomy and reasons actually exist and make sense.

If Benson's and Westlund's claims are solid, and if the critique conducted in this chapter holds, then autonomy requires conditions that cannot be captured by the monological framework. To resolve the contradictions of internalism, we must not only move beyond the dichotomy of internal and external reasons but also – and more importantly – abandon the monological conception of the agent.

Both Giordano and the MCA adopt a monological view of autonomy. The MCA assumes that individuals are so ideally disconnected from the world that they can still be autonomous even when their conclusions appear irrational. Giordano, accepting this idea as true, argues that it should be extended to patients with anorexia. Yet, examining the constitutive values of internalism shows that many of the MCA's contradictions stem from an inarticulate and clumsy commitment to the value of autonomy.

In order to overcome such contradictions and to develop a conception of mental capacity responsive to anorexics' reasoning, it is necessary to abandon the monological conception and radically rethink autonomy, taking into account the relational constitution of the agent. This is, in short, what I shall do in the remaining part of this book.

4

Relational Autonomy and Monological Agents

Building on Charles Taylor's insights, I have argued that internalist conceptions of autonomy lead to contradictions because they are rooted in a *monological framework*. In this view, agents are seen as possessing *absolute epistemological independence* – securing both their *exclusive* self-transparency and their capacity to judge values and reasons from a purely neutral point of view. These 'monological' agents are imagined as detached from the world, like self-contained systems, able to act autonomously even when their actions appear irrational, because the basis of their actions is accessible only to themselves. As Diana Meyers points out, internalism fails to acknowledge its own value commitments. It presents itself as value-neutral, obscuring its underlying dedication to a particular conception of autonomy. To address this contradiction, I argue, we must rethink autonomy beyond the monological model and instead recognize the relational constitution of human agency.

In what follows, I examine the debate on relational autonomy to assess whether – and to what extent – relational approaches might still retain elements of the monological framework. After exploring several feminist accounts of relational autonomy, I will focus on two core tensions that shape this debate: first, the role of oppression and human vulnerability; and second, the distinction between *causal* and *constitutive* models of relational autonomy.

Relational autonomy: Genesis and basic questions

Between the late 1970s and the 1990s, feminist scholars such as Lorraine Code[1] and Alison Jaggar[2] offered wide-ranging critiques of the concept of autonomy. These critiques share the conviction that 'it is certainly true that the earliest feminists were inspired by the liberal ideal of autonomy [but also that] the liberal conception of human nature and of political philosophy cannot constitute the philosophical foundation for an adequate theory of women's liberation'.[3] Code, for instance, argued that autonomy was tied to a view of the person shaped by masculine ideals of self-sufficiency and instrumental rationality, conflating 'autonomy with individualism'.[4] As a result, this concept positioned interdependence and care as incompatible with the atomistic life of the autonomous individual.

This was not just a theoretical issue. In societies marked by gender inequality, women are often expected to be primary caregivers, making it harder for them to achieve autonomy as traditionally defined. More deeply, individualism clashes with the feminist understanding of people as socially embedded, vulnerable and subject to discrimination. Neither Code nor Jaggar rejected autonomy outright. Instead, they called for a reconfiguration of the concept – one that could account for the impact of oppressive contexts on the effective exercise of autonomy.

In 2000, the edited volume *Relational Autonomy* by Catriona Mackenzie and Natalie Stoljar brought together scholars engaged in this rethinking of autonomy. The book aimed to challenge 'the conviction that the notion of individual autonomy is fundamentally individualistic and rationalistic' and to 'draw on aspects of the feminist critique of autonomy to reconceptualise and refigure the concept of individual autonomy from a feminist perspective'.[5]

Relational theorists argue that autonomy is not at odds with the idea of a relational, interdependent and socially situated agent. Scholars of relational autonomy, as well as other philosophers,[6] claim that interpersonal relations and social contexts are *necessary conditions* for the development and maintenance of agents' autonomy:[7] not only do we learn what it means to be responsible and able to choose within particular sociocultural contexts, but we also develop and shape our identity, desires and values, in accordance or disagreement with others.[8] Moreover, the exercise of autonomy depends on a network of social structures – including people, values, norms, institutions and common goods[9] – that cannot be taken for granted.

In this framework, protecting autonomy involves more than shielding individuals from *direct* interference.[10] It also requires attention to the many *indirect* ways that social relations and contexts affect a person's ability to act autonomously. Relational theorists argue not only that the concept of autonomy is compatible with feminism but also that it is essential for articulating two fundamental and intertwined ideas of contemporary feminist philosophy: the relational constitution of the agent and the systemic nature of social oppression.[11] The feminist idea of a socially embedded agent seeks to explain how, to what extent and under what conditions individuals can live according to their values and reasons in social contexts that are inimical to self-government and self-determination.

One of the paradigmatic questions relational theorists address is this: how can we distinguish between women who authentically choose to conform to subordinate roles imposed by society and those whose choices are shaped by oppression?[12] The literature on relational autonomy does not offer a single, unified answer, but scholars agree that this question cannot be resolved – or even properly formulated – without engaging with the concept of autonomy.[13]

The answers proposed by relational theorists generally fall into two broad categories: those aligned with a *procedural* conception of autonomy and those rooted in a *substantive* conception. According to procedural conceptions, the capacities for self-governance and self-determination do not depend on the content or outcome of an agent's choices but rather on their ability to apply a *correct procedure of thought* in evaluating their preferences, motives and desires. While procedural theorists differ on what constitutes a valid procedure, they commonly affirm that autonomy can be exercised even under conditions of social oppression – and that it is possible, under certain conditions, to authentically choose to conform to subordinate roles.

By contrast, substantive conceptions hold that autonomy depends on the compatibility of individual choices with a set of 'good' values and reasons. Substantive theories also come in different forms, commonly distinguished as *strong* and *weak*. Strong substantive conceptions claim that certain actions or decisions are, by definition, excluded from the domain of autonomy due to their content. Weak substantive theories, on the other hand, connect autonomy to certain relational and self-regarding capacities – such as the disposition to 'hold herself answerable, for her action-guiding commitments, to external critical perspectives',[14] or with a set of self-regarding attitudes such as self-respect and self-worth.[15]

While weak substantive theories preserve a degree of value-neutrality – since they do not evaluate autonomy based on the 'rightness' or 'wrongness' of decisions – they nonetheless affirm that specific interpersonal capacities and self-regarding attitudes are necessary conditions for autonomy. Both strong and weak substantive theories emphasize that oppressive contexts can undermine autonomy. However, whereas strong theories are more inclined to see oppressive contexts as fundamentally incompatible with autonomy, weak theories maintain that while choices made under such conditions are suspect and merit close scrutiny, they may still be autonomous.

Procedural approaches emphasize the agent's capacity to achieve autonomy even in unjust conditions; substantive approaches stress the ways in which oppressive relational contexts can impair autonomy. Both are motivated by a central concern of feminist theory: the structural and often invisible nature of oppression. From a relational standpoint, oppression is not limited to overt, intentional domination by one group over another. Rather, it is understood as a complex, diffuse set of sociocultural dynamics – embedded in norms, practices, institutions and language – that serve to sustain and perpetuate social inequality and injustice.[16] As Veltman and Piper write:

> Oppression presents multiple faces, including marginalization, exploitation, and powerlessness, and extends beyond economic and political forces to include psychological barriers that reduce, limit, or mold people as members of certain groups.[17]

Oppression is not an external interference upon an otherwise neutral or free social space; rather, it is an integral part of the social context itself. Even when it does not directly impair the autonomy of the oppressed, its indirect effects can be decisive for the development and exercise of the capacities associated with autonomy. Classical examples of the indirect implications of oppression are the phenomena of *adaptive preference formation*[18] and *internalized oppression.*[19] In these cases, individuals living under oppressive conditions may come to desire what is in fact oppressive to them or cease to desire what is denied to them, reshaping their preferences in accordance with what they perceive as their available options.[20]

Proponents of substantive conceptions of autonomy typically argue that agents who adapt in this way cannot be considered autonomous,[21] as their desires reflect an internalization of oppressive norms rather than an expression of self-governance. Procedural theorists, by contrast, acknowledge that such phenomena may signal a potential failure of autonomy but maintain that their mere presence is not sufficient to conclude that autonomy is absent.[22]

Despite these differences, both approaches share a core assumption regarding the relationship between autonomy and oppression: to understand autonomy, one must attend to the social context in which it is developed and exercised. Conversely, analysing the phenomenon of oppression requires a focus on the concept of autonomy, since one of the defining features of oppression is its tendency to undermine or erode agents' capacities for self-governance.

On oppression

As we have just seen, relational theorists have different perspectives on autonomy and on the relation between oppression and the agent's capacity to self-govern. Relational autonomy literature does not offer a unified account but, as Mackenzie and Stoljar underline, a *family* of accounts:

> The term 'relational autonomy', as we understand it, does not refer to a single unified conception of autonomy but is rather an *umbrella term*, designating a range of related perspectives. These perspectives are premised on a shared conviction, the conviction that persons are socially embedded and that agents' identities are formed within the context of social relationship and shaped by a complex of intersecting social determinants, such as race, class, gender, and ethnicity. Thus, the focus of relational approaches is to analyse the implications of the intersubjective and social dimension of selfhood and identity for conceptions of individual autonomy and moral and political agent.[23]

At a basic level, all scholars agree that oppressive social contexts can impair autonomy – at least with regard to the development of the capacities associated with it. The general assumption is that oppression *can* damage autonomy. However, there is significant disagreement about the *specific conditions* under which this potential becomes effective.

Advocates of *strong* substantive conceptions of autonomy argue that motivations formed within, and in accordance with, oppressive contexts are incompatible with genuine autonomy. Marina Oshana, for example, claims that 'the practical control autonomy demands draws both from sources internal to the agent and from external authority of a variety that mandates the absence of domination'.[24] Similarly, Natalie Stoljar maintains that a relational account of autonomy must include the idea that 'preferences influenced by oppressive norms of femininity cannot be autonomous'.[25]

In her discussion of Kristin Luker's *Taking Choices*[26] – a study of women who took contraceptive risks during the 1970s – Stoljar contends that the women interviewed were 'overly influenced in their decisions by stereotypical and incorrect norms of femininity and sexual agency' and that 'women who accept [these norms] accept something *false*'.[27] According to Stoljar, these women made decisions – such as not using contraception – based on reasons that are inimical to women's autonomy and ultimately grounded in falsehood. Some feared that using contraception would signal a premeditated sexual life and thus an improper familiarity with premarital sex. Others adhered to cultural or religious norms that prohibited contraception. Still others hoped that pregnancy would increase their perceived desirability, affirm their femininity, compel a partner to formalize the relationship or gain attention from others.

In Stoljar's view, the issue lies in the internalization of false and oppressive norms. Women who accept such norms lose the ability to recognize their *falsity* and, consequently, are unable to reflect rationally on the decisions shaped by them. Oppressive norms are, in this perspective, fundamentally incompatible with autonomy because they occlude the moral and epistemic insight necessary for self-governance. However, the mere fact that an agent endorses a false or socially constructed norm does not necessarily mean they are incapable of exercising autonomy. The role that such a norm plays in their identity, in their deliberative process, and in relation to other beliefs and commitments cannot be determined solely by the content of the norm itself.[28]

For this reason, both proceduralists and weak substantivists have offered critiques of strong substantive conceptions. Scholars such as Meyers[29] and Christman[30] argue that agents can exercise autonomy even under oppressive conditions. Paul Benson[31] has also warned that strong substantive theories incorporate a notion of morality essentially conflated with autonomy that could lead to paternalistic interventions. Indeed, one of the primary shortcomings of strong substantive accounts is their lack of nuance: they struggle to distinguish between cases in which oppression truly undermines autonomy and those in which it does not.

Defenders of *procedural* conceptions of autonomy present a position that stands in sharp contrast to the views advanced by Oshana and Stoljar. They argue that actions grounded in oppressive norms do not necessarily lack autonomy, provided those norms are *reflectively endorsed* by the agent. John Christman, for example, asserts that 'insofar as a person has authentically embraced even (what we might call) oppressive social status or subservient roles, that person deserves respect insofar as her judgment about those roles has the same formal features as our own judgment about our own lives'.[32] According to Christman, a decision is autonomous if the agent regards it as *her own*,[33] and if they have not resisted – or would not have resisted[34] – the process and context through which the motivational set underlying that decision was formed.[35] These criteria, along with the agent's ability to consider and weigh alternative courses of action, are sufficient – on Christman's account – to establish the proper functioning of her reflective capacities and thereby her ability to self-govern and self-determine.[36]

> [The reflective capacities of an autonomous agent] must contain sufficient flexibility that she could imagine responding appropriately to alternative reasons (where 'appropriately' and 'reasons' are understood from her own point of view). Adequate reflection requires that a person can see herself doing otherwise, under at least some imaginable conditions; otherwise she is not manifesting a true capacity to consider her own internal states.[37]

From this perspective, oppressive conditions are not *a priori* incompatible with autonomy, because agents can adopt a point of view in which these conditions appear preferable – even when compared with alternative reasons. If an agent is capable of reflecting on their motivational set, if that set has been – or would have been – developed without resistance, and if they are able to weigh alternative options, then they are autonomous. On this view, there is no justification for impeding or questioning their choices, even if those choices ultimately undermine or devalue their capacities for self-determination and self-government. Thus, Marilyn Friedman, a proponent of content-neutrality and proceduralism, argues that professional caregivers should refrain from trying to persuade abused women who choose to remain in abusive relationships – *provided* their decision is self-reflective.[38] Like any other autonomous agent, she contends, these women deserve professional, *uncritical* support for 'whatever choices they make'.[39]

This position appears deeply problematic to defenders of substantivism.[40] For agents living in oppressive contexts, the reflective processes they engage in may be shaped by adaptive preferences or internalized oppressive norms. These norms and preferences are often perceived by the agent as authentic; they do not necessarily obstruct reflection on alternative options, but they do make alternatives seem less desirable than those aligned with the oppressive framework the agent has internalized. The 'appropriateness' of reflection on alternative reasons, as well as the authenticity of the motivational set, cannot be adequately evaluated from the perspective of the agent alone – particularly when such reflection rests on false assumptions or is limited by a restricted availability of practicable options and perspectives. Nonetheless, for Christman and other proceduralists, the content of the motivational set is irrelevant, so long as the agent is capable of reflecting reflect – in their terms – on their decisions and on the norms that they accept.

Put plainly, proceduralist and substantivist theorists diverge sharply in how they respond to the question: *can an agent autonomously choose oppression?* Oshana and Stoljar answer in the negative; Christman and Friedman in the affirmative. Yet, despite the deep heterogeneity – and sometimes outright opposition – among the various accounts collected under the umbrella of 'relational autonomy', there are three key assumptions that justify grouping them into a coherent philosophical field.[41] These are:

A. Oppression can impede the development and the exercise of autonomy.
B. While the traditional notion of autonomy is entangled with masculinist and individualist ideals, it remains a vital concept for articulating emancipation. However, the concept must be reconfigured to acknowledge human vulnerability and interdependence, rather than presupposing self-sufficiency, independence and perfect rationality as defining traits of the autonomous agent.
C. Agents are embodied and socially, historically and culturally embedded. Their identities and capacities cannot be understood apart from these contextual frameworks.

All accounts of relational autonomy share these three assumptions, though only in broad and general terms. As we have seen, assumption **A** – that oppression can impair autonomy – is interpreted in markedly different ways depending on how the relationship between oppressive contexts and agents' autonomy is conceived. Substantive accounts maintain that oppression can distort both the decisional process and the identity of the agent, thereby undermining autonomy. In contrast, procedural accounts focus primarily on defending the agent's capacity to reflect, decide and act on the basis of their own reasons and motives, even when those reasons emerge within – and are shaped by – an oppressive environment.

On vulnerability and dependence

Regarding point **B**, relational theorists agree that the norm for human agents is not to be self-sufficient, entirely rational, or in 'full possession' of their capacities. Rather, they emphasize that vulnerability, interdependence and reliance on the practical availability of goods, care and opportunities are fundamental features of the human condition. However, relational theorists diverge in how they define and conceptualize this vulnerability and interdependence.

Seeking to offer a flexible and inclusive characterization of vulnerability – one that can accommodate a wide range of perspectives – Mackenzie, Rogers and Dodds write:

> Human life is conditioned by vulnerability. By virtue of our embodiment, human beings have bodily and material needs; are exposed to physical illness, injury, disability, and death; and depend on the care of others for extended periods during our lives. As social and affective beings we are emotionally and psychologically vulnerable to others in myriad ways: to loss and grief; to neglect, abuse, and lack of care; to rejection, ostracism, and humiliation. As sociopolitical beings, we are vulnerable to exploitation, manipulation, oppression, political violence, and right abuses.[42]

Since this notion covers a broad range of human vulnerabilities, Mackenzie proposes dividing it into two subsets, based on their source.[43] On the one hand, humans are *inherently* vulnerable due to their bodily existence; on the other, they are susceptible to a *context-dependent* form of vulnerability that Mackenzie calls *situational*.[44]

Inherent vulnerability refers to the fact that, regardless of context, we are shaped by the fragility and mortality of our bodies, along with our material and caring needs. In *Dependent Rational Animals*, Alasdair MacIntyre connects this dimension of vulnerability to autonomy. He argues that it is a mistake to assume that the capacity to make autonomous choices is disconnected from our embodied existence, since this assumption obscures the bodily and animal aspects of human rationality. According to MacIntyre, the human capacity of being rational cannot be completely separated from our animality: 'we remain animal selves with animal identities',[45] and despite the differences between other animals and humans, 'we never separate ourselves entirely from what we share with them'.[46]

Thus, our ability to reason and choose, then, is inseparable from the conditions of our bodily and animal existence: vulnerability, affliction, dependence, disability, aging and death. Many philosophers – especially within the empiricist-liberal tradition – have treated these conditions as accidental, unrelated to 'true' rationality.[47] But for MacIntyre, this view distorts the nature of human reasoning and neglects the role of relationships. A key thesis of *Dependent Rational Animals* is that the capacities for rationality are bound up with the capacities to recognize and respond to vulnerability and care:

> The virtues of independent rational agency needed for their adequate exercise [are] accompanied by … the virtues of acknowledged dependence, [so] that a failure to understand this is apt to obscure some features of rational agency.[48]

Mackenzie and MacIntyre both argue that autonomy can't be properly understood without acknowledging that the capacities for choice and self-governance are exercised by humans who are *inherently* conditioned by their bodily and relational existence. As MacIntyre puts it, 'Acknowledgment of dependence is the key to independence.'[49]

Humans are inherently vulnerable because they need food, shelter, care, social interaction and opportunities to develop and exercise autonomy. These needs, rooted in our bodily condition, make our capacities fragile – always exposed to disruption, decline or loss. Still, while some vulnerabilities are inescapable, they don't affect everyone equally. They depend on individual bodily constitution and sociocultural circumstances. To account for this, Mackenzie introduces the concept of *situational vulnerability*. It highlights those aspects of human life that 'may be caused or exacerbated by personal, social, political, economic, or environmental situations'[50] and that are connected to a wide 'range of factors, such as age, gender, health status, and disability'.[51] Unlike inherent vulnerability, situational vulnerability captures conditions that may be short-term, intermittent or long-lasting:

> For example, a person who has just lost his job is situationally vulnerable. This vulnerability may be short-lived if he has educational qualifications and skills that are in demand in the marketplace. But if the loss of a job leads to long-term unemployment, his vulnerability may be enduring and its consequences quite catastrophic, resulting not only in loss of income but also possibly loss of secure housing, marital breakdown, and ill health.[52]

Losing a job, for instance, can trigger short-term vulnerability but also lead to deeper, lasting vulnerability. It may cause depression, fatigue, low energy and difficulty concentrating or making decisions. Conversely, some forms of inherent vulnerability increase the risk of situational vulnerability: someone with depression may struggle to find or keep a job.

Humans are not only inherently vulnerable – they also need care and support to develop and exercise autonomy. Self-governance depends on a broad network of social relationships, institutions and access to resources. Oppressive relations and unjust norms can hinder it. For this reason, Mackenzie claims that 'the obligations arising from vulnerability extend beyond the *protection* from harm to the provision of the social support necessary to *promote* the autonomy of the persons who are 'more than [inherently] vulnerable'.[53] This is a key point: a relational focus helps reveal the impact of norms and institutions on vulnerability. Policies can indeed worsen inherent vulnerability or create new situational ones, rather than promoting the development and exercise of autonomy.

Relational theorists agree that protecting vulnerable individuals must go hand in hand with promoting their autonomy.[54] But they differ over which kind of autonomy to promote, and which forms of vulnerability or types of agents require support. While most agree that an approach to vulnerability grounded in the enhancement of autonomy limits the possibility that 'vulnerability may be used to sanction unwarranted paternalistic forms of intervention',[55] the boundary between supporting autonomy and being paternalistic is not fixed, and an intervention considered supportive by one theorist might be viewed as coercive by another.

These differences often reflect the divide between procedural and substantive accounts. Proceduralists, who see autonomy as compatible with oppressive norms, tend to favour value-neutrality and minimal intervention. Substantivists, who view oppression as incompatible with autonomy, are more open to relational values and interventions that help create the conditions for self-governance. Ultimately, the interpretation of assumption C – that agents are socially, historically and culturally embedded – is central. It shapes how A and B are understood (the role of oppression, and of vulnerability and interdependence in autonomy), and more broadly, how relational autonomy itself is defined.

On the necessary conditions for autonomy

In the literature on relational autonomy, differences in how the relational nature of agents is understood are often expressed through the distinction between *causal* and *constitutive* conceptions. According to causal views, social, cultural and historical contexts have a direct impact on the *development* of the capacities associated with autonomy, but they are not a constitutive part of its defining conditions .[56] From this perspective, social relationships are preconditions for *developing* autonomy, but not for *exercising* it: 'Social relationships are merely causal conditions that are required for autonomy but are no part of what autonomy specifically *is*.'[57]

Constitutive (or intrinsically relational) views disagree. For these theories, contexts do not pertain *only* to the development of the capacities of self-government and self-determination, but also to their *maintenance, enhancement* and *exercise*.[58] In this view, social contexts and relationships are constitutive parts of autonomy, no less than the individual to whom autonomy is attributed. As I will argue, this approach is the most promising for addressing the complexities of anorexia and autonomy in a sensitive and non-discriminatory way.

Procedural theories tend to be *causally* relational: they hold that once developed, the agent's reflective capacities remain functional even within unjust or oppressive contexts. After acquiring self-reflection through social support and cultural input, the agent can continue exercising it independently. Substantive theories, by contrast, are usually constitutively relational: they argue that 'a person's ability to be a self-governing agent is a function of that person's socio-relational status'.[59] On this view, autonomy does not depend exclusively on the agent's reflective capacities, but also on factors ascribable to the social, cultural and relational frameworks in which the agent acts.[60]

This distinction between causal and constitutive views marks one of the most irreconcilable divides within relational autonomy theory. It's not only a matter of how much weight to give to social context, but a disagreement over the very concept of *human agent*. Causal views see individuals as ultimately able to act independently of their formative social environment. Constitutive theories insist that relationships, culture and history remain central to autonomy throughout life – not just in its development, but in its exercise and endurance.

Relational and monological?

Causally relational accounts see autonomous agents as *epistemologically independent* from the social contexts they inhabit.[61] Within this framework, agents who conform to subordinate roles or follow self-defeating beliefs are acting on *their own reasons*. Becoming autonomous, here, means learning to manage a private domain of self-chosen norms and acting in line with individual preferences. As long as the agent reflects on these preferences and follows their own reasons and values, their capacity for self-government is not to be questioned – regardless of how much their decisions may seem to undermine autonomy.

This view of human agency clearly draws on an internalist conception of reasons.[62] Internalism appeals to relational theorists because of its supposed normative neutrality: autonomy is seen as a matter of correct self-reflection, regardless of what the agent reflects on. Consequently, autonomous agents are free to decide for themselves without being constrained by any moral requirement. This perspective on the agent is not – at least not explicitly[63] – committed to any particular conception of 'good'; it does not prescribe any action for given contexts; it avoids paternalism and supports pluralism of reasons and values. But, as we've seen, internalism's claim to neutrality is misleading. Its foundation rests on a particular set of values,[64] even if unacknowledged. This oversight leads to a superficial understanding of the role of values and reinforces an atomistic picture of the individual.

So, we must ask: can a causally relational theory of autonomy still be called 'relational' if it adopts an atomistic view of the agent and an internalist account of reasons? I've shown that internalism is tied to a *monological* view of the agent. Causally relational theories treat agents as epistemologically and morally independent from their social context – yet they also hold that agents require specific social frameworks to become autonomous in the first place.

More precisely, autonomy doesn't emerge in just *any* social setting: it depends on a context where autonomy is practiced, taught and culturally supported. Agents learn to be autonomous because others, already embedded in such a framework, *introduce* agents to activities and social practices involving the exercise of autonomy. But if agents are fundamentally detached from others and if reason is just instrumental, they can develop autonomy only if there are individuals who – using the monological lexicon – are *motivated* to introduce pre-autonomous agents to autonomy. This means autonomy is sustained only by individual, *contingent* preferences. Neither individuals nor society is intrinsically committed to promoting autonomy. Within an instrumental logic, the fact that someone is autonomous offers no reason in itself to protect or support their autonomy.

Causally relational theories define themselves as 'relational' because they see autonomy as socially developed. But their understanding of the agent implies that autonomy is not developed *through* society, but rather *in spite of it*, through individual motivations. Can we really call such a theory 'relational' if it treats society as a set of subjective, relativistic ends?

Insofar as I think theories should avoid structural inconsistencies, I frankly think they cannot. A theory of autonomy that limits the role of relations to a developmental phase ends up relying on a radically individualistic and self-sufficient model of the agent – one at odds with the non-individualist vision claimed by both relational and feminist theorists. As Charles Taylor argues,

> Social freedom is based on the notion, first, that developed freedom requires a certain understanding of self, one in which the aspirations to autonomy and self-direction become conceivable; and second, that his self-understanding is not something we can sustain on our own, but that our identity is always partly defined in conversation with others or through the common understanding which underlies the practices of our society … The identity of the autonomous, self-determining individual requires a social matrix, one for instance which through a series of practices recognizes the right to autonomous decision.[65]

According to Taylor, the role that relational contexts play for autonomy pertains both to its *causal, temporary limited* functions and to its *intrinsic, ongoing* aspects.[66] Society, relations, culture and history are all conditions of the existence of agents' autonomy, not only in terms of its development but also, and more fundamentally, in terms of its *exercise* and *sustenance*. As Taylor emphasizes, agents form their identity through dialogue with others, shaped by shared (or conflicting) practices, values and ideas. Their ability to self-govern depends on the roles they hold (or are expected to hold) in relationships, on how they see themselves, and on the beliefs, preferences and values that society and culture make available for them.[67] Ignoring these dimensions would be a serious mistake for any theory that wants to be truly relational – or, more broadly, for any account of autonomy that aims to be solid, grounded in reality and non-discriminatory in practice.

Monological agents and procedural interpretations

As we've seen, relational theorists broadly agree on three points: (1) oppression can undermine autonomy; (2) autonomy needs to be rethought in light of human vulnerability; and (3) agents are socially embedded. I've shown that these assumptions are interpreted differently across theories, dividing mainly into two camps: proceduralist and substantivist (or three, if we distinguish strong from weak substantivism). These interpretations are linked: how one understands (1) and (2) depends largely on how (3) is framed. Some take (3) to mean that agents need relationships to *develop* autonomy (the causal view), while others see relationships as shaping the *exercise* of autonomy itself (the constitutive view). I've critiqued the causal view for being incompatible with the non-individualist vision of the agent upheld by feminist and relational thinkers. Now, I'll turn to how proceduralist interpretations of (1) and (2) are tied to a monological reading of (3). This step will help refine which relational views of autonomy genuinely respond to feminist critiques of individualist models.

From the point of view of the relation between oppression and autonomy, proceduralism differs from substantivism in claiming that agents can autonomously choose subservience or endorse oppressive norms. Marilyn Friedman writes:

> Women [who are] motivated to stay in abusive relationships by questionable normative commitments … are living their lives in accord with norms that are evidently very important to them … On content neutral accounts of autonomy, these women might well qualify as autonomous … On these

> accounts, someone is autonomous as long as her choice meets certain non substantive criteria, such as being the result of reflection on her deeper values and commitments … Someone's self-reflections and choices under [coercive] conditions are less likely than otherwise to be reliable reflections of what she really cares about. Yet it is not impossible to discern or act according to one's deeper concerns under coercive conditions.[68]

For Friedman, an agent's decision to accept coercion can be autonomous if they reflectively endorse a set of motivations, preferences, values and beliefs that make that decision seem worthwhile. Christman agrees, adding that the agent's motivational set and evaluative structure must be *authentic* and *historically* (or autobiographically) grounded, that is, they must be 'seen as *mine*'[69] and accompanied by a critical reflection on the historical processes surrounding their development.[70] In short, autonomy can be exercised in oppressive contexts if three conditions are met:

1. the agent has sufficient self-reflective capacities;
2. their motivational is authentic;
3. they did not – or would not – resist how the motivational set was formed.

What stands out in these conditions is their content-neutrality: autonomy is judged by formal features of the agent's reasoning, not the content of their motivations. If someone acts according to a motivational set they see as their own, they are considered autonomous. It does not matter that a decision is autonomy-devaluing and based on oppressive values if the procedure of thought applied by the agent reflects their identity in a way that is acceptable *for them*. In one of his articles, Christman writes:

> We must coordinate our acts and reasons with others, either by being called on to account for our actions and values in ways that force us to reflect on them or by listening to the reflections of others in acting with them or in response to them. But *deliberate action for the self-governing agent* may well be passionate, committed, unflinching, and hence *nonreflective* in any given instance. This does not mean, however, that such action is unthinking or not underwritten by one's basic values (often quite the contrary). But it

> does mean that in acting one engages the value orienting function of one's practical identity and in so doing reaffirms that identity as worth having and acting upon.[71]

Christman argues that autonomous decisions can be made regardless of the relational context. This is a typical causally relational leitmotiv: once autonomy is developed through relations, agents 'obtain' the capacity to disengage from them and act solely based on self-determination. But this is no accident. Proceduralist theories are *necessarily* tied to a causally relational perspective. Their refusal to assess the content of an agent's values can be justified only on the ground of agent's capacity to self-determine their motivational set independently of the relational context.

When proceduralists say 'oppression can interfere with autonomy', they really mean 'oppression can interfere with the *development* of autonomy'. The first two procedural conditions – self-reflection and authenticity – are not truly relational. Agents acting on private values they see as authentic are deemed autonomous, even if their motivations are shaped by oppressive norms. The third condition – the agent's non-resistance to how their motivations developed – might seem relational, but it only refers to the past – when the basis for autonomy has been laid – not the actual exercise of autonomy in the present.

As I've argued, views on how oppression affects autonomy depend on how one interprets relational embeddedness. Proceduralism relies on a causally relational model, which assumes a monological agent and conflicts with feminist ideas of vulnerability, interdependence and social embeddedness. It also struggles to address internalized oppression and adaptive preferences. As Paul Benson points out, oppressive norms can become so ingrained that it's unreasonable to claim agents could – or would – have resisted the formation of autonomy-limiting preferences:

> Feminine socialization gains much of its power by operating to deceive many women about the significance that cultivating an appearance which is pleasing to men has for women's worth as persons. Women's autonomy is reduced to the extent that they are socially trained to be blind to the reasons there are for them to regard their appearance differently than the norms of femininity recommend.[72]

Internalized norms and adaptive preferences pose a challenge to autonomy precisely because individuals accept them as their own, without resistance.[73] Agents can form autonomy-limiting motivational sets because they live in contexts where accepting oppressive norms or subordinate roles is often necessary – even required – to be seen as worthy.[74] These unjust norms obscure the reasons an agent might have to resist them, making the issue both deeply complex and ethically urgent.[75] As Christman notes, some agents 'who never cave in to the oppressiveness of their conditions either by losing their oppression-independent self-understanding or by losing their will to resist'.[76] But this doesn't mean that those who don't resist – or wouldn't have resisted – are autonomously choosing conformity. On the contrary, as Benson stresses, the lack of resistance can itself be a result of life within an oppressive context, where unjust values become internalized and preferences adjust to a limited set of options defined by unfair norms.[77]

In a nutshell, procedural theories are grounded in a causally relational conception of autonomy, and thus in a monological view of the agent. This means that although they acknowledge relational conditions for the development of autonomy, they ultimately treat agents as atomistic individuals who self-govern in ways that can be opaque or inaccessible to others. I've already discussed the flaws of this view, but let me add one more. Because of their monological conception of the agent, proceduralists are inclined to see forced intervention as a *justified violation* of liberty – paternalism – that is, as an act that is justified but that is also intrinsically violent and coercive. This framing shows a limited understanding of the vulnerable and interdependent nature of human beings. As Mackenzie argues, this proceduralist commitment to non-interventionism (or negative consideration of intervention) implies an underestimation of social injustice and vulnerability, placing the burden not on institutions or social structures but on the individuals themselves:[78]

> If autonomy is understood relationally, the apparent opposition between responding to vulnerability and promoting autonomy dissolves. Indeed, from the perspective of a relational account of autonomy, although the duties arising from vulnerability include protection from harm, the duty to protect must be informed by the overall background aim of enabling the development of, or fostering, autonomy whenever possible.[79]

Conceptions of autonomy that rely on a monological view tend to frame intervention as justified interference aimed at defending autonomy, rather than as a collaborative act of care intended to build or restore the conditions for autonomy's development and exercise. As Mackenzie notes, a relational lens avoids conflating intervention with a violation of liberty by reframing both personal and social responsibilities and by blurring the line between promoting autonomy and responding to the different forms of vulnerability that affect agents.

If my argument holds, proceduralist accounts and causally relational notions of autonomy suffer from the same issues as the monological framework they rely on. Like that framework, they fail to secure the value-neutrality they claim to offer, and they do not provide a meaningful set of conditions capable of addressing the concerns raised by relational autonomy. Moreover, monological conceptions are characterized by insoluble epistemological issues.

To overcome the limitations of proceduralist and causally relational accounts, we need to rethink relational autonomy with close attention to the conception of the human agent it presupposes. This agent cannot be monological. It cannot be seen as exercising self-determination independently of relational contexts or as unaffected by the structural presence of oppression and inequality in society. The concept of autonomy must rest on a view of the human agent as shaped, embedded and constituted by non-ideal relational contexts – contexts marked by systemic injustice and social dynamics of domination.

If this line of analysis and strategy is right, what will emerge is a richer, more fine-grained conception of autonomy – one grounded in a broader and more realistic account of human agency. This, in turn, will enable us to encompass, grasp and address the specific issues affecting the troubled relationship between anorexia and autonomy, finally allowing us to approach the central problems of this book with a whole new set of analytical tools.

5

The Conditions of the Exercise of Autonomy

reframing neutrality: Inescapable values and autonomy

The debate on relational autonomy unfolds along three main axes: the substantiveprocedural axis (S/P), the causal-constitutive axis (C/C), and the value-neutral/value-laden axis (N/L). In Chapter 4, I introduced the first two. Here, I return to my critique of value-neutrality by focusing on the third.

A theory's position on the N/L axis depends on whether it includes values among the conditions required for autonomy. This axis allows for no degrees – only a typological distinction: either values are considered or they aren't. From this angle, the N/L axis overlaps with the S/P axis. Procedural theories define themselves through value-neutrality, while substantive ones focus on the content of the agent's values.

I specified that substantive theories come in *strong* and *weak* forms. Strong theories hold that certain values and preferences are inherently incompatible with autonomy. Weak theories, instead, link autonomy to dialogical capacities (like dialogical answerability[1]) and to self-regarding attitudes (like self-respect, self-worth and self-trust). This difference entails two key distinctions. First, strong substantivism excludes autonomy-incompatible outcomes by default. Weak substantivism does not predict specific outcomes but insists that certain attitudes and dispositions are required to secure agents' dialogical accountability and their status as moral and political agents.[2] Second, while strong conceptions are explicitly *value-saturated*, weak ones retain a degree of value-neutrality. Being sustained by a *particular* set of values, strong substantive theories are de facto incompatible with value-neutrality. Weak substantive notions do not assess agents' autonomy on the grounds of the compatibility of their choices with a set of 'good' values and reasons but acknowledge that certain value-related capacities and dialogical attitudes are necessary conditions of the exercise and maintenance of autonomy.

For proceduralists, a theory is value-neutral only if it ignores the content of agents' values, motives and preferences. From this standpoint, both strong and weak substantivism are value-laden and therefore disqualified from neutrality. But, as I've argued, this approach is inconsistent. As Meyers[3] and Taylor[4] point out, all theories of autonomy – whether they admit it or not – are normatively constraining and grounded in a particular set of values. A fully neutral perspective is not viable because the very act of theorizing assumes a background that privileges certain elements over others. As Taylor writes, 'We are always and inevitably thinking within such taken-as-granted frameworks.'[5] Value-neutral conceptions, moreover, are normatively internalist – and as we saw, internalism fails to deliver the neutrality it promises.

My point is that a *coherent* theory of autonomy – one that can reflect on its own moral commitments – must be, to some degree, *value-laden*. Meyers claims her account is value-neutral because autonomy can't be deduced from the values it assumes (such as self-respect or dialogical accountability).[6] But since these are treated as necessary conditions for autonomy, her account falls within weak substantivism. Given that all autonomy theories are value-based and normatively constraining, terms like 'value-neutral' or 'normatively neutral' are ultimately misleading. Finally, the divide between strong and weak substantivism shows that the value-neutral/value-laden dichotomy is poorly drawn – and unhelpful for addressing the many ways value-neutrality can be configured.

If, as I've argued, the proceduralist distinction between value-neutral and value-laden fails to capture the actual role values play in theories of autonomy, then the philosophical framework of relational autonomy needs to be rethought. In particular, we need to distinguish between coherent relational accounts and incoherent ones based on monological conceptions of the agent. To do this, I propose reconfiguring the N/L axis so that it excludes purely value-neutral approaches from the field of relational autonomy, while recognizing the different ways values can be subsumed into theory. This reworking requires two adjustments: (1) replacing the value-neutral end of the axis with an asymptote – something theories can tend towards but never fully achieve; (2) dividing the value-laden side into distinct zones, each reflecting a different mode of integrating values. For this, I refer to the categories I proposed for Meyers's Directivity Axis: value-saturated, intermediary value-laden and dialogically value-laden.

Once reconfigured, the N/L axis still tracks differences of kind, but now becomes sensitive to varying degrees of value-ladenness. Its ends are no longer 'value-neutral' and 'value-laden', but instead mark two distinct positions: value-saturated on one side, and what I propose to call *dialogical* value-laden on the other, with an *intermediary* value-laden position in between. These positions reflect different proximities to the asymptote of value-neutrality:

1. *Value-saturated* notions hold that only moral choices can count as autonomous.[7] They place clear constraints on what agents can choose and thus sit furthest from the value-neutral asymptote.
2. *Intermediary* value-laden accounts include *external* conditions like access to meaningful options[8] or freedom from social oppression. Though they don't assess the agent's values directly, they still restrict what counts as an autonomous choice by focusing on external factors – hence, they are closer to neutrality than value-saturated theories but still place a direct constraint on the content of the agent's choices and actions.
3. *Dialogical* value-laden conceptions place emphasis on relational capacities (like answerability) and self-directed attitudes (like self-worth). These theories don't limit what agents choose but rather how they relate to their reasons and values to others and to themselves – making them the closest to value-neutrality, without claiming full neutrality.

In conclusion, values and morality – just like the psychological functions emphasized by proceduralists – are built into the very concept of autonomy. While relational accounts can be more or less neutral with regard to the values and preferences endorsed by the agent, the possibility of a coherent, purely value-neutral approach is averted. A coherent conception of autonomy, in other words, requires some sort of moral background.

The necessity of language

Why does the monological conception remain attractive and widespread, despite the contradictions and issues I've analysed? In my view, the main reason is that this conception *appears* as implicitly built into autonomy itself. If autonomy means *self*-governing on the basis of one's *own* reasons and values, it appears obvious that the individual – who supposedly has *privileged* and *direct* access to these values – cannot be questioned about how to apply them. After all, we might think, nobody *else can truly know my values and reasons as I do, nor can they know better than I how to act accordingly.*

The problem, as I've argued,[9] is that the apparent validity of this reasoning is fundamentally illusory, based on unexamined assumptions. This epistemological model presumes that agents have *unmediated, privileged* access to their motivational set and that their reasons and values exist in a *private* domain accessible to others only indirectly and partially. These assumptions form the foundation of any theory of autonomy adopting a monological conception of the agent. Therefore, formulating a coherent notion of autonomy requires challenging these assumptions and rethinking self-knowledge *within* a relational framework. Let us now turn to this task. In *Philosophical Arguments*, Taylor writes:

> [The monological view] situates thought and knowledge within the mind of the individual. Of course we share things, such as bodies of knowledge and language, but these are seen as matters we converge on. It means, for instance, that my language is close to yours and to hers and to his. If I am to be a speaker, then there must be such a thing as my language, my idiolect; and if there is to be common knowledge, then it must be first of all my knowledge, and yours, and hers and his.[10]

From a monological perspective, agents can adjust their understanding to converge with others' viewpoints, enabling complex social interactions. However, this shared knowledge remains fundamentally *derivative* – formed by partial overlaps of the *original* knowledge occurring privately within each individual's mind. Agents, then, remain essentially epistemologically independent. Common knowledge, unlike individual knowledge, is always mediated, secondary and diachronically subsequent.

Explicitly or implicitly, the monological approach treats individuals as *epistemologically independent*: each has a private language and personal understanding, and linguistic interactions occur only to the extent that their private understandings coincide or align in a shared language.[11] For instance, Locke argues that the meaning of a word lies not in its relation to objects but rather in the ideas representing these objects.[12] Thus, monological epistemology grounds all knowledge in the individual's capacity to associate objects of knowledge – mental contents – with the words or concepts representing them. Yet, as Taylor emphasizes, this epistemological model leaves unexplained why mental contents should be *directly intelligible*. It simply assumes this intelligibility as an *obvious*, self-evident fact about humans, requiring no further justification.

> Proponents [of epistemological independence] suppose that a word can be given meaning in some ceremony of naming, or that its meaning can be imparted by pointing to the object it names … Naming something seems like a primitive, self-sufficient operation.[13]

The capacity to grasp the relationship between a sign and an object of knowledge – such as defining something ostensively or naming it – is seen as *preceding* and *grounding* the learning and development of language. This ability is regarded as an intrinsic human characteristic. Both Condillac's fable of the two children in the desert[14] and Augustine's account of language in his *Confessions*[15] exemplify this idea: humans *naturally* learn to interpret, for example, crying as a sign of pain, and in doing so, they acquire the first elements of their language.

Yet, this perspective is problematic and ultimately flawed. Firstly, *it presupposes what it aims to explain*, assuming humans *naturally* possess the capacity to understand something as standing for something else. Secondly, it does not explain *how* we could understand the meaning of a sign *before* having developed language itself – like someone 'came into a foreign country and did not understand the language of the country; that is, as if he already had a language, only not this one. Or again: as if [they] could already *think*, only not yet speak. And "think" would here mean something like "talk to himself"'.[16] Finally, this account does not provide any insight into human capacities for understanding and using signs that would not equally apply to pre-linguistic or non-linguistic animals.

> I have the word 'triangle' in my lexicon. This means that I can recognise things as triangles, identify them, pick them out as such. I can say, for example, 'this is a triangle'. But what does this capacity amount to? … I might train an animal (a rat), to react differentially, say, to go through a door which had a triangle painted on it, as against one which had a circle. So my rat would be in a sense recognising a triangle. But there is a crucial difference: the rat in a sense recognises the triangle, because he reacts to it. But the human language-user recognises that this is a triangle, he recognises that 'triangle' is the right word to use here; that this is the right description. This capacity to recognise that X is the right description is essentially invoked in our capacity to use language.[17]

Our capacity to recognize and to operate with signs (what Taylor, following Herder, calls *reflection*[18] (*Besonnenheit*)[19]) is different from the capacity of pre-linguistic animals because the kind of task performed by humans is *intrinsically defined in linguistic terms*, or – in other words – because only *within* language is it possible to understand something as meaningful or signifying, to understand that a sign is 'right' for a certain purpose.[20] A rat's ability to identify a triangle is assessed according to its effectiveness in achieving a non-linguistic goal (e.g. obtaining cheese). Humans, on the other hand, recognize a triangle in terms of the correctness of this recognition itself. By treating mental contents as immediately intelligible, inherently meaningful, we obscure the linguistic character of human understanding. This results in fundamentally distorted conceptions of knowledge, relations and values.

But if, as I argue, human knowledge depends on language, am I not simply restating the same problem differently? After all, if epistemological independence wrongly assumes the innate ability to recognize signs, why would highlighting the ability to recognize the *rightness* of signs be less problematic? Because, unlike the former, the latter can be *explained* rather than merely assumed. The capacity to recognize a sign as the 'right' one depends on what Taylor calls a *background*.[21] Wittgenstein's remarks in the *Philosophical Investigations* clarify this point:

> So one could say: an ostensive definition explains the use – the meaning – of a word if the role the word is supposed to play in the language is already clear. So if I know that someone means to explain a colour-word to me, the ostensive definition "That is called 'sepia' " will enable me to understand the word … One has already to know (or be able to do) something before one can ask what something is called.[22]

Wittgenstein argues that understanding an ostensive definition already presupposes acquaintance with the language within which that definition makes sense;[23] indeed, 'to understand a sentence means to understand a language'.[24] For example, to grasp that someone pointing and saying 'this is called "sepia" ' is teaching us a colour's name, we must already possess substantial contextual knowledge and familiarity with human practices. As Wittgenstein immediately adds, 'What does one have to know?' We must know that by pointing, the person refers to something (not directing attention to the finger itself), that the indicated feature is a colour (not shape or sound), and that we are learning a name (not being instructed merely to repeat a sound). We also need to understand the social practice of naming, know that colours can be named and recognize that 'sepia' refers to colours generally – not only to that specific object's shade and so on.[25] Thus, *we need to be acquainted with a whole contrastive dimension*.[26]

However, there is an intrinsic difficulty in replying to the question 'what does one have to know?' On the one hand, if taken literally, it resists a definitive answer, being poorly formulated.[27] As I will argue, what we must know can only be partially articulated, never fully. On the other hand, if we interpret the question *figuratively*,[28] answering it necessarily involves acknowledging the background's role in knowledge, thereby overcoming the assumptions of epistemological independence and monologicity. Indeed, 'what we have to know' is not simply *another* definition or *another* sign among signs.

> When we find a certain experience intelligible, what we are attending to, explicitly and expressly, is this experience. The context stands as the

> unexplicited horizon within which … this experience can be understood … [The background] is that of which I am not simply unaware, as I am unaware of what is now happening on the other side of the moon, because it make intelligible what I am uncontestably aware of; at the same time, I am not explicitly or focally aware of it, because that status is already occupied by what it is making intelligible. Another way of stating the first condition, that I am not simply unaware of it, is to say that the background is what I am capable of articulating, that is, what I can bring out of the condition of implicit, unsaid contextual facilitator – what I can make articulate, in other words. In this activity of articulating, I trade on my familiarity with this background. What I bring out to articulacy is what I 'always knew', as we might say, or what I had a 'sense' of, even if I didn't 'know' it.[29]

Thus, human knowledge rests upon a background that remains structurally *unsaid*. The success of an ostensive definition like 'this is "sepia"' relies fundamentally on the listener's ability to pragmatically infer a broad range of implicit assumptions, all taken for granted.[30] As Wittgenstein emphasizes, the inarticulateness of the background is not due to contingent limitations, speaker incompetence or deficiencies in language itself.[31] Although the background can be partially articulated, it remains inherently impossible to fully describe, since any articulation itself depends on what the background already makes intelligible. As Wittgenstein argues, 'It is not [through] ignorance. We don't know the boundaries because none have been drawn … We can draw a boundary – for a special purpose. Does it take this to make the concept usable? Not at all! (Except perhaps for that special purpose.)'[32] The role of the background is to make our linguistic operations possible, to make certain experiences intelligible.[33] Consequently, the background can be only *partially* articulated, and solely for specific purposes – just as I am attempting here[34] – because

> we can never fully dominate [the background]; and yet we are never fully dominated by it, because we are constantly reshaping it. Reshaping it without dominating it, or being able to oversee it, means that we never fully know what we are doing to it.[35]

Against relativism and private language

This inquiry brought us here: the basic assumption underlying epistemological independence – the idea that humans instinctively understand their mental contents – is unfounded. As Wittgenstein and Taylor argue, self-knowledge depends on language, which itself relies on a broad network of capacities, practical know-how and familiarity with human practices – what Taylor calls a *background*. Language cannot be described simply as correlations between words (utterances) and things (mental states),[36] nor as a finished product or set of ready-made instruments. Language is primarily a *pattern of activities*,[37] within which the ability to designate things is just *one* among many tasks we perform. Through language, humans continuously 'recreate, extend, alter, and reshape'[38] language itself, along with the forms of awareness, knowledge and expression that it allows. Yet, as Taylor remarks:

> If language must be primarily seen as an activity, if it is what is constantly created and recreated in speech, then it becomes relevant to note that the primary locus of speech is *in conversation* … Language is fashioned and grows not principally in monologue, but *in dialogue*, or better, *in the life of the speech community*.[39]

Taylor's and Wittgenstein's views of language (which I call *dialogical conception*) fundamentally challenge monological epistemology. Shared knowledge is neither *derived* from nor secondary to self-knowledge; rather, *language is an irreducible dialogical activity*. Therefore, the realm of rightness, truth and falsity – the fundamental kind of human knowledge that distinguishes us from animals – cannot be private but must be common. This reverses the monological view: we can grasp mental contents only because we first learn – or, rather, inherit[40] – a language in which this possibility is realized.

Before moving forward to explore the implications of the dialogical conception for autonomy, I want to clarify two key points for my argument:

1. A radical dialogical conception avoids the relativism and subjectivism of the monological framework. More precisely, it is intrinsically opposed to such philosophical drifts.

2. The dialogical conception rules out the possibility of private languages or purely private mental content.

Let me explain. A common misunderstanding of the so-called 'late' Wittgenstein concerns his view on agreement, particularly agreement in judgements, as foundational for knowledge and language. Since Wittgenstein claims that knowledge happens within language, which is a dialogical activity shaped by a largely unarticulated background, it might appear that he is saying 'that human agreement decides what is true and what is false'.[41] On the contrary,[42] Wittgenstein clearly argues the opposite: human agreement depends on objective conditions, including our bodily, embedded and interdependent nature – what he calls a *form of life*.[43] As Wittgenstein himself puts it:

> What is true or false is what human beings *say*; and it is in their *language* that human beings agree. This is agreement not in opinions, but rather in form of life. It is not only agreement in definitions, but also (odd it may sounds) agreement in judgements that is required for communication by means of language. This seems to abolish logic, but does not do so – It is one thing to describe methods of measurement, and another to obtain and state results of measurement. But what we call 'measuring' is in part determined by a certain constancy in results of measurement.[44]

Wittgenstein uses an analogy between language and measurement to clarify why his view does not undermine logic.[45] He explains that describing a measuring method and actually using it are distinct operations, each with different goals and functions. First, the former relies on the latter: in order to describe methods of measurement, we must be able to use a method of measurement.[46] Without the ability to measure – without *any* method of measurement – we would lack criteria to distinguish or describe measuring methods at all.

Second, the concept of 'rightness' involved in each case is different. When we use a measuring method, its 'rightness' depends directly on achieving our practical aim.[47] In contrast, the 'rightness' of describing a measuring method depends on the criteria we apply when analysing descriptions.[48] Yet neither the 'rightness' of the description nor the method itself can be entirely detached from the practical act of measurement. Simply put, a measuring method is 'right' if it achieves its goal effectively, and a description is 'right' if it helps ensure better, more consistent or sufficiently precise measurements (or avoids worse, inconsistent or imprecise ones).[49]

When Wittgenstein speaks of an 'agreement in judgement' in human knowledge, he means that everyone who knows how to measure practically agrees on what constitutes a consistent measurement. But this agreement in judgement is not mere opinion or arbitrary consensus. Even though our understanding of 'measurement' does not assume some ideal consistency, perfect method or universally objective standard, this does not imply the abolition of logic or absolute freedom to define measurement however we like. Rather, our definition of measurement is shaped – at least partly – by the efficacy of our habits and by the results of our acts, which are in turn regulated by the conditions set by our bodily, relational and environmental conditions. Grounding rightness in human agreement does not eliminate logic; it only removes the expectation of logic's 'crystalline purity'.[50] As Wittgenstein writes, 'One might say: the inquiry must be turned around, *but on the pivot of our real need.*'[51]

In short, relationality implies neither relativism nor subjectivism. It is not human agreement that decides what is true or false; rather, truth depends on our practical realities: the things we do or avoid doing, the actions we cannot help performing, our bodily existence, the environments we inhabit, our dependence on others and their dependence on us. The agreement underlying language and knowledge is *internal* to our dialogical practices – *it is an agreement in our form of life.* Although this agreement cannot be fully articulated or described externally, it remains neither arbitrary nor subjective.[52]

For similar reasons, the possibility of a *private* conception of language or mental contents is ruled out. Knowledge always takes place within language, and language is inherently dialogical, grounded in non-arbitrary shared activities that constitute our form of life. Consequently, the very idea of a private language, along with a private, purely personal knowledge of one's mental contents, is incoherent. Locke's affirmation, 'every man has so inviolable liberty to make words stands for what ideas he pleases',[53] turns out to be blatantly wrong. Wittgenstein captures this clearly:

> Suppose that everyone had a box with something in it which we call a 'beetle'. No one can ever look into anyone else's box, and everyone says he knows what a beetle is only by looking at *his* beetle. – Here it would be quite possible for everyone to have something different in his box. One might even imagine such a thing constantly changing. – But what if these people's word 'beetle' had a use nonetheless? – If so, it would not be as the name of a thing. The thing in the box doesn't belong to the language-game at all; not even as a *something*: for the box might even be empty – No, one can 'divide through' by the thing in the box; it cancels out, whatever it is.[54]

The metaphor of the beetle in the box illustrates the inconsistency of assuming private, direct knowledge of mental contents. If we suppose that no one else can look inside our box, and we cannot look inside theirs, the actual *content* becomes irrelevant to how we talk about the boxes. The legitimacy of our statements about the boxes remains independent of what they contain; whether they have a beetle, a die or nothing at all changes nothing.[55] Wittgenstein's aim is not to deny that personal or internal objects (such as reasons, values, motives and sensations) exist but to highlight, first, that these objects are not private[56] and, second, that the meaning of what we say about them is *structurally independent of their content*. In short, the content of 'what we have in mind' is ultimately *irrelevant* to the meaning of 'what we have in mind'.[57] 'What we have in mind' is, like all meanings, embedded in the dialogical activities through which language articulates meaning. As Cora Diamond puts it, 'What objects we are thinking about is something that is shown in the language we use.'[58]

In this section, I have shown how a dialogical conception of knowledge can overcome the structural problems inherent to monological epistemology while avoiding the pitfalls of relativism and subjectivism. Moreover, recognizing the role of values and reasons in knowledge opens conceptual space for examining the relationship between morality and the necessary conditions for autonomy. In the next section, I shall explore this conceptual space further, focusing especially on the role values play within the dialogical framework and examining more closely the relationship between weak substantivism and relational autonomy.

The dialogical conception and relational autonomy

At this point, we must return to the monological assumptions and consider the implications of a dialogical conception for autonomy. Doing so will allow me to reformulate the idea of self-knowledge *within* a dialogical framework and to propose a constitutively relational conception of autonomy capable of overcoming the limitations identified in this book.

One of the reasons the monological framework remains so appealing, despite its contradictions, is that it seems inherently connected to the concept of autonomy itself.[59] If autonomy means self-governance according to one's own reasons and values, it is *somehow obvious* that the *owner* of those reasons and values must not be impeded in applying them. Since individuals supposedly have *direct*, *privileged* access to their reasons and values, they alone seem capable of genuinely knowing and applying them. Yet, as I've argued, these assumptions are mistaken. Humans neither possess direct, privileged access to their mental states nor truly 'own' their reasons and values. Following Taylor's and Wittgenstein's insights, meanings are dialogically constituted – both in their origins and in their ongoing conditions of existence. Thus, it is erroneous to speak of privileged access to meaning, whether considered 'internal' or 'external', as meaning always operates within language, which is inherently dialogical and public.

The idea of direct knowledge is fundamentally misleading,[60] as it implies the existence of objects of knowledge separable from their contexts and conditions of existence. Additionally, it suggests that this knowledge could be practically infallible. But as Taylor and Wittgenstein have demonstrated, language is a pattern of activity that does not accommodate infallibility.

Finally, humans do not *own* our reasons and values. As shown in Chapter 3, values and reasons are neither purely internal nor external; they are not located solely 'in the mind' or 'out there'. More aligned with the perspective of this book, values and reasons constitute and are part of[61] the *background* of human activities – they constitute the *contrastive* and *logical* space within which we operate as linguistic and political beings. Humans can 'have' reasons and values because language allows them to do so. What it means to 'have reasons and values' is never fixed once and for all but always dependent upon the dialogical context within which such expressions gain their significance. As Wittgenstein puts it:

> 'Following a rule' is a practice. And to *think* one is following a rule is not to follow a rule. And that's why it's not possible to follow a rule 'privately'; otherwise, thinking one was following a rule would be the same thing as following it.[62]

Applying and understanding one's reasons and values must be recognized within the background in which we act as bodily and dialogical beings. Acknowledging the role and significance of this background is crucial for autonomy. By clarifying the conditions that underpin language and knowledge, we can specify some necessary – but not sufficient[63] – conditions for self-understanding and autonomous action. The dialogical approach developed in this book presents an account of self-knowledge that is structurally relational and inherently situated within a dialogical and embodied framework. According to this perspective, the objects of self-knowledge are not private or isolated but integrated into a shared language. Autonomous agents act within a background in which these possibilities are pragmatically contemplated and judged as *important*.[64]

Constitutively relational autonomy and weak substantivism

The dialogical framework I'm outlining aligns with a constitutive approach to autonomy: relationality is integral to autonomy's defining conditions. The capacity to self-govern and self-determine is not only relationally developed but also – and more fundamentally – *relationally exercised*. In broad terms, autonomy inherently depends on conditions beyond the agent's individual capacities or psychological faculties:[65] to act autonomously, agents must be embedded in a relational context that affords the possibility of their autonomy *and* that makes this possibility intelligible.

At this stage, it is reasonable to suggest that theories describing *irrational* or *ungrounded* decisions as autonomous[66] contain inconsistencies. To act autonomously, agents must satisfy relationally grounded moral and rational criteria. But what are these conditions? Before addressing this, I want to introduce a distinction to avoid potential misunderstandings. Relational theorists commonly distinguish *global* from *local* conceptions of autonomy:[67] global autonomy refers to the conditions defining the agent's capacity 'to exercise authentic, reflective self-control over extended portions of one's life',[68] while local autonomy refers to autonomy concerning specific actions or decisions.[69] I will not engage with global autonomy here for three reasons. First, my purpose is to address a *specific*, problematic case of autonomy assessment.[70] Second, I agree with Christman that agents can 'display all the level-headedness and freedom of thought characteristic of autonomy'.[71] For example, a person with a phobia is unable to self-govern only in those contexts involving their phobic triggers. Lastly, a global conception clashes with my aim to highlight autonomy's situated and dialogically dependent characteristics: from the perspective of embodied, relationally embedded agents – who are inherently vulnerable, fallible and interdependent – a strictly 'all-or-nothing'[72] conception of autonomy appears inconsistent and idealistic.

Keeping in mind this local approach, what relational conditions qualify an agent as autonomous? Based on my analysis thus far, we know these conditions must (1) take into account the content of the agent's motivational set; (2) be based on values that do not directly constrain the agent's choices and outcomes; and (3) represent necessary but insufficient conditions for autonomy.[73] Adopting relational theorists' terminology, we could say these relational conditions belong to *weak substantivism*, a theory connecting autonomy with dialogical attitudes, values and dispositions that do not predetermine agents' outcomes. Advocates of weak substantivism have explored these conditions by following two partially interconnected approaches: first, by examining agents' self-regarding attitudes such as self-worth, self-respect and self-trust; and second, by considering the role of dialogical answerability and recognition. In the next section, I shall examine these two approaches in order to understand whether, and to what extent, they fulfil the three criteria outlined earlier.

Self-regarding attitudes: Self-worth, self-respect and self-trust

As we have seen, some conceptions of autonomy are more value-neutral than others, yet it remains logically impossible to offer a *fully* value-neutral account of autonomy. The notion of autonomy is already value-laden. Take, for instance, the concept of a 'promise': its meaning is inherently tied to a moral framework, and it cannot be reduced to purely value-neutral terms without extracting it from the background in which a promise makes sense. At a fundamental level, to speak about autonomy is to speak about something *intrinsically important*. The significance of autonomy is part of its very meaning. Thus, we can understand *recognizing* the value of autonomy as a prerequisite for its exercise.[74] Autonomous agents see themselves as *worthy* of taking responsibility for their lives and of acting on their values and reasons; agents who do not view themselves as valuable cannot genuinely engage with their values and reasons as worthy of expression or defence. Without this self-valuing background, how could an action even be considered an *act* at all? How could we distinguish it from *behaviour*?

In my critical discussion of internalism,[75] I introduced Paul Benson's concept of self-worth, referencing his example of the gaslighted woman. Benson asks us to imagine a woman who 'arrives at her sense of incompetence and estrangement from her conduct on the basis of reasons that are accepted by a scientific establishment which is socially validated and which she trusts'.[76] According to Benson, even if this woman acts reflectively, she cannot be considered autonomous because she lacks a 'sense of [her] own worthiness to act, or of [her] status as agent'.[77] Or, as Mackenzie puts it, she 'will think that who she is or what she does makes no difference, and hence she will think that she will have no motivation for resolving internal conflicts, for trying to establish a reflective equilibrium among the different elements of herself'.[78]

Benson highlights two important points here: first, agents may become disconnected from their reflective capacities due to insufficient self-worth;[79] second, procedural conditions alone are not sufficient for evaluating autonomy. Rather, it is essential to consider the value agents assign to themselves and thus examine the content of their motivational set. Importantly, despite proceduralists' objections, examining self-worth in a substantive way does not necessarily lead to paternalism or violate value-neutrality. Assessment of self-worth cannot foresee what an agent sure of their self-worth will decide in a specific context, nor prescribing any 'adequate' course of action.

As Benson and other relational theorists emphasize, self-worth is fundamentally 'sensitive to others' attitudes toward the agent';[80] in other words, self-worth is partially dependent on relational recognition. Even though self-worth is a *self*-regarding attitude, it should not be seen as independent from others: on the contrary, self-worth depends significantly on how others perceive and value us, directly or indirectly, through social and cultural expectations related to gender, race, ethnicity, social status, disabilities, religion or sexual orientation. Self-worth is developed and maintained within relational frameworks, which vary greatly in how they attribute worth to agents based on factors – such as gender, ethnicity or social background – that have nothing to do with the agent's actual worth. From this perspective, the connection between oppressive contexts and autonomy becomes clear in ways proceduralist and causally relational accounts fail to capture: by attributing lesser value to certain agents, oppressive contexts create dialogical conditions that may erode the self-worth of those agents who are normatively devalued. Oppression is not in itself a sufficient condition for heteronomy;[81] yet, given how crucial others and social contexts are for developing and exercising self-worth – and therefore autonomy – it is important to carefully assess the self-worth of people embedded in normative and relational contexts that have historically undermined their worth as agents.[82]

Robin Dillon argues that self-worth is not only a necessary condition of the exercise of autonomy but also for the development and sustainment of *self-respect*. Self-respect, in turn, constitutes a further requirement for the exercise of autonomy.[83] According to Dillon, self-respect coincides with many aspects with self-worth – included its relational constitution – yet it is not limited only to the recognition of the 'person's status as a full and equal member of the moral community and as the bearer of certain basic moral rights' but also involves the recognition of one's own inherent vulnerability and dependence:[84]

> A feminist recognition of self-respect would … involve two other attitudes: acceptance and patience. For insofar as respecting myself entails acknowledging the extent to which I am always in transition, always under construction, it will require patience. And insofar as I am limited, imperfect, liable to failure and to fragmentation and incoherence, insofar as the details of my life will include much that is not admirable or lovable or nice, self-respect will require a deep and abiding acceptance of myself that goes beyond toleration.[85]

A person with self-respect is to some degree able to acknowledge and accept her vulnerable, fallible and dependent nature. She adopts an attitude towards herself that involves self-care and rejects self-neglect and self-abnegation.[86] However, this does not mean self-respect includes indiscriminate self-acceptance, self-indulgence or self-obsession. In fact, these attitudes are incompatible with self-respect,[87] because the self-respecting agent engages in a caring relationship with themselves and others that involves the recognition of their own vulnerabilities.

Self-worth and self-respect are not the only dialogical self-regarding attitudes taken into account by theorists of relational autonomy: scholars such as Trudy Govier,[88] Carolyn McLeod[89] and Susan Sherwin[90] argue that a certain degree of *self-trust* is also a necessary condition of the exercise of autonomy. As McLeod and Sherwin write:

> Exercising autonomy involves, in part, reflecting on one's beliefs, values, and desires: making reasonable decision in light of them; and acting on those decisions. It is essential in developing the capacity to be autonomous that the agent trust her capacity to make appropriate choices, given her beliefs, desires, and values; that she trusts her ability to act on her decisions; and also that she trusts the judgments she makes that underlie those decisions … Without trust in the judgments and trust overall in her ability to exercise choice effectively, any agent would have little motivation to deliberate on alternative courses of action.[91]

McLeod and Sherwin argue that the conditions self-trust sets for autonomy are threefold:[92]

1. the agent must trust her capacity to act in accordance with her values and reasons;
2. the agent must trust that she can effectively act on her decisions;
3. the agent must trust the judgments behind her decisions.[93]

Without the first condition, an agent distrusts her own decision-making abilities or doubts whether she properly understands the relevant facts. She struggles to articulate her beliefs and desires clearly. Without the second condition, an agent doubts her ability to practically realize her decisions, becoming uncertain about her reliability as an agent. An agent lacking the third condition questions her own judgements about her decision-making process, undermining confidence in her ability to form motivations responsive to her identity. Given the relational nature of knowledge and language, it is incorrect – as relativists or subjectivists might argue – to say that agents who lack self-trust simply 'trust their distrust'. Self-trust applies only when an agent sees herself as trustworthy, capable of acting according to her values, reasons and judgements, actively engaging with her decisions.

McLeod explicitly frames self-trust as a self-regarding *moral* attitude:[94] 'All autonomous decisions have a moral aspect; and therefore, self-trust can be the self-regarding attitude that motivates us to be autonomous. In choosing and acting autonomously, we strive to meet moral responsibilities to the self, to others, or to both.'[95] Recognizing autonomy's moral dimension does not lead to paternalistic or biased interventions, as proceduralists fear. We can't predict exactly what decisions an agent with self-trust will make, but we can ensure these decisions satisfy the conditions of existence of autonomy.

Like self-worth, self-trust depends partly on the relational context in which the agent is embedded, influencing both its development and exercise.[96] However, unlike self-worth, self-trust connects to the reliability and epistemic status of an agent's capacities and must be *justified* to some extent. As Govier argues, 'One may have more confidence in one's own character and capacities than past experience and evidence would warrant, thus having "too much" self-trust in an epistemic sense … [Or] even supposing that evidence and experience warrant one's confidence in oneself, one may rely on oneself so much that one precludes potentially valuable contributions from others.'[97] Thus, 'the relation between self-trust and autonomy is reciprocal, not unidirectional'.[98] Autonomy depends on self-trust, but self-trust also requires autonomy and adequate knowledge for justification. For example, I shouldn't trust myself to fly an airplane if I lack the necessary skills. A person with unjustified self-trust will most likely be impermeable to external critiques and considerations, so their autonomy would not be sustained by an adequate degree of dialogical answerability.

Having explored these self-regarding attitudes, I now turn to another value central to weak substantivism: dialogical answerability.

Dialogical answerability and recognition

Dialogical conditions of autonomy are not limited to self-regarding attitudes but also involve the agent's disposition towards interaction. Andrea Westlund argues that an autonomous agent must 'hold herself answerable, for her action-guiding commitments, to external critical perspectives'.[99] Proceduralists stress critical reflection but often underestimate how relational factors influence its application and sustainability.[100] Even if an agent believes her choices reflect her authentic commitments, without openness to critique 'practical reasoning will be strangely disconnected from, and insensitive to, any justificatory pressures to which she, the agent, is subject'.[101]

What is meaningful for human agents, their 'dimension of meaningfulness', is relationally constituted: agents do not possess a private language or grasp their own thoughts in isolation. Rather, agents develop and shape their identities, as well as their values and reasons, in interaction and in contrast with others. 'An agent who holds herself answerable for her action-guiding commitments effectively shows that, however firmly committed she is to certain values, she is not just passively in their sway.'[102] Consequently, agents who are not able or willing to interact with other critiques and considerations prove not to be actively engaged in the dialogical process of defence and revision of their motivational set; or, to put it bluntly, they are partially inoperative in relation to the activity of reflection itself.

Westlund's account of autonomy, like McLeod's, Benson's and Dillon's, is weakly substantive.[103] She argues that dialogical answerability does not place direct normative constraints on agents' decisions or motivations but only indirect constraints on their dialogical attitudes and capacities. Martha Nussbaum challenges this view, claiming dialogical answerability and self-regarding attitudes might restrict certain choices, such as genuine religious commitments based on external authority.[104] However, Nussbaum's objection misunderstands dialogical conditions: dialogical accountability and self-regarding attitudes are not 'inconsistent per se with religious commitment, but it is inconsistent with dogmatic forms of religious commitment, or any other form of dogmatism, for that matter, which involve appeals to authority that bypass a person's reflective agency'.[105] In order to be dialogically answerable the agent does not have to endorse or reject any particular belief and preference but has to participate in the social activity of articulation, testing and – eventually – modification of one's own identity[106] – a kind of activity that, as we have seen, is necessary for self-understanding.[107]

Since answerability is relationally constituted, it depends significantly on the dialogical context. This implies two things: first, oppressive conditions can undermine an agent's disposition towards answerability; second, the relational context itself must remain responsive to the agent's creative or potentially *subversive* contributions. Let me expand this point. It is impossible to predict precisely what autonomous agents will choose, how they might embody cultural norms or when those norms might obstruct their autonomy. Autonomous agents often conflict with existing relational contexts, articulating their autonomy by challenging and transforming prevailing norms. Women who fought for the right to vote in the early twentieth century, for example, exercised and articulated their autonomy in the political sphere by conflicting with the normative structure in force.

As a consequence, not only can autonomous agents enter into conflict with their relational context, but also be, as a result, unable to exercise their autonomy without *altering* the current norms of the relational context in a way that makes their claim recognized and articulable. Agents do not simply and passively 'follow the rules'; their relational constitution does not prevent them from changing what constitutes them. On the contrary, agents can come to alter the norms of the relational context by making their dissent dialogically intelligible, proposing alternatives and clarifying why certain norms impede autonomy. Here it becomes crucial to stress that the relevance of dialogical answerability to autonomy does not affect only the agent but also the normative structure itself: if the relational context does not contemplate the possibility that agents can have something reasonable and unpredicted to say regarding the normative structure, something that can have *effective* consequences on the normative structure, then the agents' attitude to dialogical answerability can be impeded, neutralized or *put into crisis*. If society is unjust, short-sighted or simply unwilling to recognize how its norms affect the autonomy of some agents, then it is reasonable for those agents who are oppressed and not heard to disobey the established norms. Stanley Cavell describes very well the latter circumstance in *Conditions Handsome and Unhandsome* in relation to Henrik Ibsen's *A Doll's House*:[108]

> In *A Doll's House* the thematics of Nora's climactic charges against her husband, Torvald Helmer, put the social order as such on notice, deploying, enchaining, amongst others, the concepts of conversation, education, happiness, becoming human, fathers and husbands, brother and sister, scandal, becoming strangers, fitness for teaching, playtime, honor, the miracle of change, journey or departure, the bond of marriage. The tone of her charge, while within the bonds of decorum due the man whose children she has borne and whose life she has shared is colored by her outburst, 'I could tear myself to pieces'. She is outraged, dishonored, ashamed … But when Nora tries to show this to Torvald he replies that she is talking like a child, that she does not understand the world she lives in (with which she agrees and which is an essential part of her determination to leave this husband and their children), … and when Nora says to Torvald, 'I must find our which is right – the world or I', he replies, 'You're ill, Nora – I almost believe you're out of your senses' … When Torvald, in a fit of ultimate blindness and self-congratulation, tells Nora that he forgives her (instead of begging for her forgiveness), she thanks him and leaves; he follows

> her to the door from beyond which, at this questioning her, she tells him she's taking off her fancy clothes; whereupon he resumes expatiating on the genuineness of his forgiveness and her need of it as he paces outside her door, stopped only as she reappears. 'What's this? Not in bed? You've changed your clothes.' And Nora replies, 'Yes, Torvald, I've changed.'[109]

In contrast to Benson's example of the gaslighted woman, Nora's self-worth remains intact despite accepting her husband's negative judgements. Although Nora agrees with Torvald that she doesn't fully understand the world around her, she never loses sight of herself as a worthy person deserving autonomy. She preserves her self-respect and self-trust, eventually leaving the oppressive relationship. Nora's autonomy is profoundly challenged within the relationship: Nora's autonomy is at stake in the relation: she is unbearably close to losing any sense of her contact with society (she agrees with Torvald that she does not understand the world she lives in) and with herself ('I could tear myself to pieces'), yet this struggle doesn't prevent her from seeking recognition and expressing her perspective to Torvald.

Nora's disposition towards dialogical answerability is severely strained because Torvald is unwilling or unable to genuinely listen. Her reasons are considered unacceptable because they are in contrast with the normative structure of the marriage, and the reasons Nora receives from Torvald are not responsive to her view of the relation and of herself. As Stanley Cavell notes, 'Specific wrong may not be claimable; yet the misery is such that, on the other side, right is not assertible; instead, something must be shown.'[110] In leaving Torvald, Nora does not only inaugurate a new life but also shows him something:[111] 'Yes, Torvald, I've changed.'

Even when Nora realizes Torvald can't – or won't – recognize her suffering as a form of oppression, she does not abandon dialogue. Instead, she gives Torvald an opportunity to understand that her oppression stems from their relationship's constraints, and that his view about her 'was not based on his judging for himself, and bearing responsiveness to his judgment, but on the imagination of rules that, as it were, replaced his judgment.'[112]

Nora's situation highlights an important aspect of dialogical answerability. If we accept that *both* agents *and* relational contexts are never ideal, and if we recognize that oppression is an intrinsic, often invisible, sociocultural dynamic connected to a set of unquestioned norms, then three points become crucial.

First, we must pay close attention to the actual dialogical responsiveness of whoever holds greater authority in the dialogue, especially when the dialogue aims to assess the other's dialogical capacities. Second, it is essential that those with authority genuinely engage with the reasons offered by others – even when they imply the subversion of current norms and particularly when these reasons imply the subversion of current authority. Finally, we must remain sensitive to the actions and expressions of agents who perceive themselves as excluded or marginalized by the relational context.

While normative frameworks cannot completely eliminate mistakes like Torvald's, they can significantly reduce such risks by adopting these precautions and fostering dialogical enrichment.[113] As Mackenzie argues, emphasizing dialogical answerability 'provides grounds for criticizing social structures as unjust and reforming them, and it provides reasons for providing targeted social support and resources to scaffold the persons' capacities for self-governance'.[114]

Having criticized value-neutral approaches to autonomy for their incoherence, I have developed a constitutive relational conception of autonomy by rejecting the ideas of epistemological independence and private knowledge and by emphasizing the dialogical constitution of language and knowledge. This enabled me to reformulate self-knowledge within a dialogical framework and to overcome the shortcomings of autonomy theories embedded in a monological perspective – specifically procedural conceptions, causally relational accounts and internalism. Furthermore, by examining the significance of self-regarding attitudes and dialogical answerability, I have clarified the functions of some key relational conditions required by my conception of autonomy.

In the next, concluding chapter, I shall return to the questions raised in the first two chapters and apply my relational conception of autonomy to the case of patients with anorexia who refuse life-saving treatment. I will assess, firstly, whether and to what extent my account can resolve the legal and ethical issues posed by anorexia, and, secondly, whether my model ultimately remains compatible with liberalism.

6

Practices of Dialogical Responsibility

After reviewing the main conceptions of anorexia, I examined the issue of anorexic patients refusing life-saving treatment, highlighting a structural problem within English law (the MCA). According to the MCA, patients must be considered autonomous until proven otherwise and permitted to refuse life-saving treatments. However, in cases involving anorexic patients, judges adopt an unusual stance, assuming – based solely on the anorexia diagnosis – that patients lack decisional capacity.[1]

I agree with Giordano that this discriminates against anorexic patients,[2] but I disagree with her *brave claim* that the MCA's requirements sufficiently assess mental capacity, making anorexics' refusals valid and legitimate. People with anorexia – particularly if unsupported – can become controlled by anorexia, losing their capacity for autonomous reflection on their decisions in ways that the MCA's procedures fail to detect. In short, the core issue of anorexic patients' lack of capacity is not tied to brain function or psychological abilities but rather to how they engage with their identity, morality, beliefs, motives, and values.

Paradoxically, the form of autonomy recognized by the MCA and defended by Giordano – leading one's life according to private motivations – is not only attained by anorexic patients, but *mastered* by them. From a 'purely' value-neutral perspective, anorexics exemplify ideal self-governance and self-determination: they do what they deem right, overcome significant physical and relational barriers to achieve their goals and remain deeply resistant to external criticism. Indeed, even though extreme advocates of value-neutrality would likely reject this conclusion, in 'purely' value-neutral terms, individuals with anorexia *are* paradigms of autonomy.

Resistance to assessing mental capacity through the content of an agent's motivational set relies mainly on three arguments. The first is value-neutrality, according to which adopting substantivism would imply prescribing specific values, thereby opening the door to authoritarianism and paternalism. However, I have shown this argument to be unfounded since every conception of autonomy inherently depends on certain values. Unlike strong substantivism, weak substantivism involves values that do not predetermine the outcomes autonomous agents will pursue, beyond the pursuit of autonomy itself.

Moreover, given the vulnerable and interdependent nature of human agents, we need a conception of intervention sensitive to the ways individuals influence and depend on one another. Intervention should not be depicted as a justified violation of liberty – a necessary, but violent and coercive act – but as supportive action responsive to relational needs.

Finally, I argued that both procedural–value-neutral and substantive–value-laden accounts fail to address the genuine difficulties presented by patients with anorexia who refuse treatment. This inadequacy stems directly from their shared monological framework, in which agents appear as isolated entities able to self-govern and self-determine in ways legitimately unintelligible to others. And if we assume agents are epistemologically independent, intervention inevitably becomes *interference* to be minimized. Yet epistemological independence is a mirage, and its underlying monological conception of autonomy contradicts the fundamentally vulnerable and dependent condition of human agents.[3] Under such a framework, intervention is confined solely to cases of malfunctioning or absent autonomy, inevitably forcing a shift towards 'best interests'.[4]

The monological framework is unable to adequately consider agents' relational embeddedness and their vulnerable, interdependent nature. Even worse, not only is it unable to take account of the role that social inequalities and injustice have for autonomy, but it also, more or less passively, perpetuates them. For these reasons, I maintain that the monological framework must be rejected. Only through adopting a dialogical perspective can we see that intervention does not necessarily constitute an intrusion into autonomy. This is true not only because interaction is integral to human life but also because intervention can enhance and promote autonomy. Thus, intervention is not justified violence, but a practice of *relational responsibility* aiming at protecting and improving autonomy.

The dilemma of patients with anorexia refusing treatment does not stem from the limited choice between two problematic options: avoiding intervention (risking abandonment) or intervening (risking violating autonomy). Indeed, the distinction between paternalism and neutrality itself rests on the false assumption that one can genuinely avoid intervention and leave the agent free to decide alone.

Where does this leave us? It appears we face the central dilemma of anorexic patients refusing treatment: relational responsibility is *inescapable*, but also *fallible*. As Sullivan and Niker write, 'The wrong of certain interpersonal intervention (when they are wrong) is not that they violate our autonomy, *but that they fail or harm us in some other way*.'[5] If this is correct, the primary question regarding anorexics' refusal is not 'should we intervene?', but rather '*how can we best intervene*?' Dialogical responsibility should not be obscured by inconsistent claims to value-neutrality. Instead, two key elements must be considered to minimize the risks of harmful interventions:

1. *The assessment of mental capacity must include the values and reasons ascribable to weak substantivism.* These values and reasons are as essential to autonomy as the functional capacities proposed by proceduralism. Their evaluation does not prescribe specific courses of action, nor does it significantly undermine value-neutrality.
2. *The autonomy of the agent cannot be separated from their relational context.* Relations are necessary conditions both for developing and exercising autonomy. This is especially true for patients with anorexia: psychiatrists, people with anorexia and former anorexics commonly underline that it is very uncommon for anorexic individuals to adopt a negative or non-egosyntonic view of anorexia in solitude. Typically, anorexic patients come to recognize anorexia as a mental disorder rather than a beneficial lifestyle or expression of their authentic self through interactions with others.

In the next two sections, I shall discuss the roles played by self-regarding attitudes and dialogical answerability in assessing mental capacity in anorexic patients who refuse treatment. I will pay special attention to highlighting and addressing the potential risks linked to weak substantivism, particularly regarding dialogical answerability. My proposals, far from being definitive, aim to indicate how to *avoid* the temptation to pursue the ineffective solutions offered by proceduralism and value-neutrality.

Self-regarding attitudes beyond self-esteem

Psychiatrists and psychologists have examined the role of self-esteem in the development, persistence and recovery from anorexia.[6] Denise Kästner and colleagues define self-esteem as 'an evaluative view of the self in its totality ... [that can be considered as a synonymous of] self-evaluation, self-respect, self-confidence, and self-worth'.[7] Similarly, Anna Brytek-Matera describes self-esteem as 'an individual judgement of advantages expressed in attitudes which are affected by humans, such as acceptance, love, self-respect, self-confidence and belief in one's own abilities'.[8]

Typically, studies on anorexia do not separately examine the roles of self-trust and self-respect, nor do they distinguish these clearly from self-esteem. As Tafarodi and Swann underline, psychiatric research often conflates self-esteem with related attitudes, referring interchangeably to 'self-esteem', 'self-competence', and 'self-liking'.[9] They define self-competence as 'the overall sense of oneself as capable, effective, and in control',[10] which aligns closely with the concept of self-trust discussed previously. Self-liking, on the other hand, refers to the 'affective judgment of ourselves', that is, 'our approval or disapproval of ourselves'. This is similar to the idea of self-worth analysed earlier, though conceptualized here within a monological framework. According to Tafarodi and Swann, 'self-liking is the *part* of self-esteem that is clearly socially dependent'.[11] Being the *part* of self-esteem that is socially dependent is obviously opposed to that element of self-esteem that is socially *independent*. Instead, I propose that self-esteem is best understood as a subcategory or synonym of self-worth, clearly distinct from self-respect and self-trust. To effectively link psychological and psychiatric studies on self-esteem with my analysis of self-regarding attitudes, I will use a more precise definition of self-worth rather than the broad notion of self-esteem employed by anorexia researchers. Specifically, I refer to Benson's dialogical definition of self-worth as the 'sense of one's own worthiness to act, or of one's status as agent'.[12] Additionally, I shall explore the distinct contributions of self-trust and self-respect.

Self-worth is widely recognized as a central factor in the onset, persistence and recovery from anorexia across major studies.[13] Fairburn and colleagues argue that all eating disorders share a specific relationship between self-worth, food intake, weight and body shape.[14] This relationship can form a vicious circle: restricting food intake and losing weight initially enhances self-worth,[15] but over time, the increasingly demanding conditions necessary to maintain self-worth become unattainable, transforming into a source of self-hatred.[16] In some cases, people with anorexia restrict food because they feel undeserving: '*I don't feel I deserve* [to eat] ... *I don't feel I deserve nice clothes. When my sister died I thought it should have been me.*'[17] Given its close relationship with anorexic symptoms, I refer to this particular configuration as *egosyntonic self-worth*. Overcoming egosyntonic self-worth and developing a non-anorexic form of self-worth is an essential step in treatment. The dissolution of egosyntonic self-worth, as well as the development of a non-anorexic form of self-worth, is a necessary step in the treatment of the disorder.[18]

Other scholars have proven that lack of self-worth is a fundamental maintenance factor of anorexia even when the lack of self-worth is not directly connected to anorexia[19] – as well as being one of its predictors[20] and relapse factors.[21] As discussed in Chapter 1, people with anorexia and post-anorexic patients consistently highlight self-worth as fundamental, agreeing on its crucial role in developing, maintaining and overcoming anorexia.

At this point, I want to address this question: what role does self-worth play when assessing anorexic patients' capacity to refuse treatment? In Chapter 5, I argued that self-worth is a necessary condition for autonomy – agents cannot autonomously make decisions unless they see themselves as worthy of making those decisions. But how does this apply to patients with anorexia? Given the multiple roles self-worth plays in anorexia, we first need to differentiate among various 'configurations' of self-worth that anorexic patients refusing treatment may exhibit. I identify four main ways in which self-worth can manifest itself:

1. *Egosyntonic self-worth*: an anorexic patient's decision can be sustained only by the kind of self-worth that accords with the symptoms of the disorder.
2. *Non-egosyntonic self-worth*: an anorexic patient's decision can be sustained by the kind of self-worth that is, at least partially, independent of anorexia.
3. *Egosyntonic lack of self-worth*: an anorexic patient can lack self-worth because she is not acting as an anorexic and because she is not starving enough.
4. *Non-egosyntonic lack of self-worth*: an anorexic patient can lack self-worth due to factors entirely independent of anorexia.

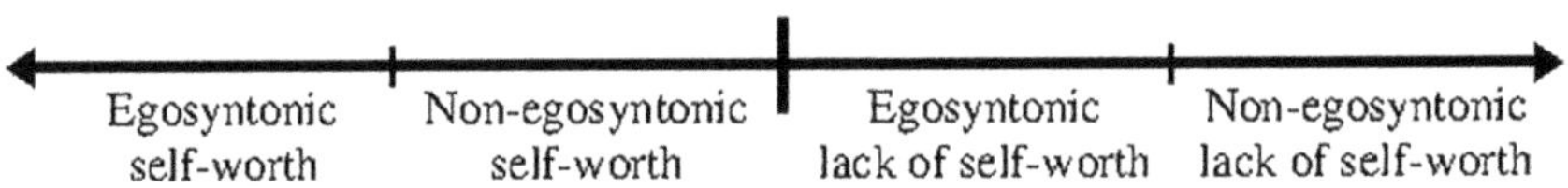

(1) highlights that self-worth can be *maladaptive*. Anorexic patients can maintain egosyntonic self-worth only by adopting a set of behaviours that are unsustainable in the long term:

Participant D: I remember getting some tests back saying how my liver was really damaged and all this, and I thought it was really rather good! I can't imagine that I thought it, it felt like really quite an accomplishment! … I'd just done something that I knew hardly anyone else could do … I can remember when I had difficulty walking upstairs, or I had such pain bending down, at the back of my legs, and I loved it, I used to bend down as much as I could to feel the pain! And I felt so in control.[22]

I think that patients with anorexia with egosyntonic self-worth should not be considered incapable of refusing treatment due to a lack of self-worth, despite its maladaptive nature. However, this does not imply that their reasons for anchoring self-worth in food restriction, body shape and weight loss are defensible or sustainable. As I will clarify in the next section, the acceptability of such egosyntonic self-regarding attitudes should instead be evaluated through the lens of the patient's dialogical answerability.

So far as I know, there is no specific literature on (2). Still, if the patient's refusal of treatment is sustained by a self-worth unrelated to anorexia, there is no reason to conclude that the patient lacks decisional capacity because of self-worth issues.

In contrast, patients who lack self-esteem (3 and 4) cannot reasonably be considered capable of refusing treatment. Regardless of the underlying reasons for their absence of self-worth, these patients lack the necessary conditions for exercising autonomy regarding treatment refusal.

But not all anorexic patients refusing life-saving treatment lack self-worth; some maintain it precisely through their anorexic symptoms. What about their self-respect? As mentioned previously, self-respect has generally received limited attention in literature and is usually conflated with self-esteem. Moreover, there are no studies specifically addressing the role of self-respect in anorexia or other eating disorders. Therefore, it is currently impossible to provide an exhaustive account of how self-respect influences anorexic patients' decisions to refuse treatment. Nevertheless, we can offer some preliminary hypotheses based on available empirical evidence.

Claudine Clucas has argued that self-respect is 'based on principled and honourable behaviour, … [and that it is] influenced by moral integrity'.[23] Following this characterization, it seems reasonable to assume, firstly, that only patients with self-worth can exhibit self-respect; secondly, that both egosyntonic and non-egosyntonic forms of self-worth can coexist with self-respect. As discussed in Chapter 1, anorexics may view anorexia not as a problem but as a lifestyle associated with distinct values, principles and morality. Many post-anorexic individuals confirm that anorexia involves complex moral and identity-related issues that persist even after treatment.[24] Finally, people with anorexia often exhibit a strong tendency to adhere strictly to extremely high standards and rigid self-evaluation criteria.[25] They can, therefore, be highly consistent in living according to their own principles and values.

Clucas's notion of self-respect could lead us to think that anorexic patients with egosyntonic self-worth can indeed have self-respect. However, we can refine this by integrating Dillon's relational condition: self-respect does not concern only the morality of the person but also the acceptance of one's own inherent vulnerability and interdependence.[26] Anorexics, especially in the early or acute phases of the disorder, can be resistant to others' critiques and refuse help entirely. Moreover, the anorexic ideal of extreme self-control appears difficult to reconcile with the vulnerable, bodily and fallible nature of human agents.

Nevertheless, there is no literature explicitly addressing the role of self-respect in anorexia or investigating how individuals with anorexia perceive their vulnerability and interdependence. Thus, it is difficult to draw fair conclusions about the role self-respect plays specifically in anorexic patients who refuse treatment. Yet, as discussed in Chapter 5, self-respect is a necessary condition for exercising autonomy, suggesting that a lack of self-respect might indicate an impaired ability to refuse treatment. Further research is therefore necessary to clarify the exact function of self-respect in patients with anorexia refusing treatment.

As with self-respect, no studies have yet specifically explored the relationship between anorexia and self-trust. However, existing literature on self-esteem, together with interviews of anorexics and post-anorexics, provides data consistent with the notion of self-trust discussed in Chapter 5. McLeod and Sherwin define self-trust broadly as applying to agents who regard themselves as deserving trust,[27] but this concept requires further clarification. Previously, we distinguished three partially interconnected forms of self-trust:

1. *Self-trust about capacities*: an agent with this form of self-trust believes they can act according to their values and reasons and that they sufficiently understand relevant information needed for decision-making. People lacking this self-trust typically express doubts such as 'I do not have control over my life', 'I don't understand what I truly want and what is right' and 'I don't know enough about this to decide'.
2. *Self-trust about the exercise of autonomy*: an agent with this self-trust believes they can effectively carry out their decisions. Typical claims made by people lacking this kind of self-trust may include 'I can't to do what I want, what is important, what is right', 'I have no control on my actions' and 'I know what I should do, but I can't actually to do it'.

3. *Self-trust about judgement*: an agent with this form of self-trust relies on their judgements as a valid basis for decisions. Those lacking commonly express 'I do not trust myself', 'My judgements are unreliable', 'I should not do what I think' and 'My decisions have no solid foundations'.

How do these notions apply to anorexia? Most patients with anorexia and post-anorexics claim that anorexia is fundamentally a way of *gaining self-control:*

Participant D:	I think [anorexia] begins with a need to control when individuals feel that various areas of their life are out of control, and they're not happy about other areas of their lives, and so they look for another way to feel in control, to feel happiness, and a way you can guarantee it is by food, by weight, by exercise.[28]
Interviewer:	You mentioned that anorexia is a symptom of something else. What is it a symptom of for you?
Rachel:	For me, I think my whole life I wanted control. And I want sameness and control and an identity and to feel accepted in some way. And I think at some point my anorexia became my identity. [29]
Participant F:	It kind of protects you as well, I think, from coping with other things. It just distracts you the whole time. Basically punishing you all day long, bullying you about something. It just fills your mind. It distracts you so completely about things you don't want to think about, to lose that is quite scary.[30]

As with self-worth, people with anorexia typically develop a maladaptive form of self-trust through restricted eating, weight control and exercise. Anorexia initially provides a comforting feeling of control and helps individuals manage identity issues, feelings of powerlessness and other personal struggles. Especially during the early or acute stages, or for those who have not undergone treatment, anorexia often offers a sense of mastery – a 'higher' and uniquely strong sense of control that appears achievable only through anorexia. Yet this reassuring sense of control usually begins to fade once the negative consequences of the disorder become overwhelming.

Participant 17: [Anorexia] is a prison, it's not just about food, it's about life I think 'cos I find that it's made me want to control everything.[31]

Participant 21: I think you feel you can control um, have extra control in your life by controlling what food you eat very, very strictly but in the end it doesn't end up you controlling it, it's kind of more it controlling you.[32]

It is very likely, then, that people with anorexia who have not yet developed a non-egosyntonic or negative understanding of anorexia may display self-trust in all three domains described by McLeod and Sherwin. These individuals have self-trust about their capacities since they believe they can govern themselves effectively and are confident about their knowledge of food, weight and exercise, as well as in their ability to apply that knowledge. However, anorexics often consider themselves exceptions to established scientific guidelines, arguing they require less food and more exercise than others, that body mass index does not apply to them, or that they are immune to the harmful effects of anorexia. This is clearly a form of excessive or unjustified epistemic self-trust, as described by Govier.[33] Nevertheless, having egosyntonic self-trust does not mean people with anorexia should automatically be considered incapable of refusing treatment. Yet, anorexics with egosyntonic self-trust should not be considered unable to refuse treatment *because* they lack self-trust. As with egosyntonic self-worth, these cases must be evaluated by examining their dialogical answerability and their capacity to respond to external critiques and considerations.

Anorexic patients with egosyntonic self-trust might also view themselves as capable of acting according to their motivational set. On the one hand, this is certainly true: anorexics are remarkably able to adhere strictly to their standards and motivations. On the other hand, individuals with anorexia experience significant challenges in acting consistently with their motivational set once they begin developing a non-egosyntonic identity and a negative conception of anorexia.

Participant 21: Well I always THOUGHT that I could, like before I tried it I thought all the time well I could easily eat more and stop this if I wanted. But when I came to try to do that I couldn't.[34]

Participant 13: When I was lying in the hospital my mum would bring over a bowl of melon and say 'Melon OK, it's just water' … I'd thinking, 'oh I really want to eat that, I want to eat, I just want to eat.' … And then when it came to it, my hands would start shaking and I'd just want to throw it across the room, I just couldn't do it, no matter how hard I tried I just couldn't physically do it … I don't even know what was stopping me, it was obviously the anorexia but my thought just changed, like one minute I would, and the next minute I just went 'NO' I couldn't do it, at all.[35]

When people with anorexia have an egosyntonic identity and a positive view of their disorder, they usually believe themselves capable of acting according to their decisions, thus showing no lack of self-worth. However, while egosyntonic traits appear reflectively endorsed by the patient, they are actually symptoms of the disorder that typically disappear after recovery. For this reason, self-trust based on egosyntonic traits cannot be considered a reliable indicator of autonomy on its own; it needs further assessment through dialogical answerability.

Lastly, individuals with anorexia who possess egosyntonic self-trust trust their judgements and believe their motivational set aligns with their authentic identity and concerns. Indeed, it is common for anorexics to perceive anorexia as their true self or as an inseparable part of who they are. Even those who experience a divided sense of self often struggle to detach from their anorexic identity and embrace their 'logical self'.

Participant 17: Quite often, people with anorexia, they don't say, 'I have anorexia', they say 'I am anorexic'. And I think that's kind of, that explains it really, that shows what it is, people BECOME anorexic, they, and then they start saying, 'I am anorexic', and it's this kind of, it becomes who you are, it defines who you are, as opposed to just an illness that you have.[36]

Participant 36: It feels like there's two of you inside, like there's another half of you, which is my anorexia and then there's the real K [own name], the real me, the logic part of me and it's a constant battle between the two.[37]

People with anorexia who require life-saving treatment are typically in the acute phase of the disorder. They will likely exhibit egosyntonic self-regarding attitudes, an egosyntonic identity and view anorexia positively. Under these conditions, an assessment might reveal adequate self-trust. However, as previously argued, having egosyntonic self-worth and self-trust does not automatically imply the capacity to refuse treatment. It remains crucial to evaluate whether their reasons for linking self-regarding attitudes to anorexic behaviours are justified or at least understandable. Since values and reasons are neither private nor comprehensible outside language and dialogue, assessing anorexic patients' dialogical answerability is central to understanding both their self-regarding attitudes and their capacity to refuse life-saving treatment.[38] Let us now explore this point, analysing dialogical answerability in anorexic patients who refuse treatment.

Refusal of treatment and dialogical answerability

I argued earlier that autonomous agents are capable, to some extent, of articulating and defending their commitments in response to external critiques. How does this apply to patients with anorexia who refuse life-saving treatment? Let's consider the case of a patient *who has never received treatment for their eating disorder*, carefully avoiding the risk – illustrated by Torvald's irresponsiveness – of imposing an adversarial dialogical framework.

The first step in assessing dialogical answerability involves determining the patient's willingness to engage with the medico-juridical assessors.[39] The assessors must clearly inform the patient about the purpose, structure and consequences of the dialogue. At this point, two outcomes are possible: the patient may accept or decline the dialogue. If the patient can articulate reasons for refusing treatment, the assessment may proceed. If they decline, it's essential to explore why they feel excluded, misunderstood or threatened by the assessors, taking their perspectives and self-narratives seriously.

If the patient accepts the dialogue, the second step involves analysing their reasons for refusing treatment and anchoring self-worth and self-trust to anorexic behaviours. The central aim of this step is to understand the *viability* of the explanations articulated by the patient, or – to put it from the point of view of the patient – to make intelligible their reasons to the medico-juridical assessors. Again, two outcomes are possible: either the patient successfully articulates their reasons – indicating dialogical answerability and capacity to refuse treatment – or they fail to make their claims intelligible.[40] The latter situation parallels the scenario discussed previously concerning the patient's initial unwillingness to engage. Let's now explore this stage more closely.

If the patient is unwilling or unable to articulate their decisions and attitudes clearly, it is necessary to seriously consider whether the dialogical setting itself is impeding their capacity for expression, or whether the assessors have insufficiently acknowledged the patient's values and reasons. Medico-juridical assessors might – like Torvald in *A Doll's House* – ground their reasoning on unquestioned assumptions structurally incompatible with the patient's claims. Consequently, some patients – like Nora – may find themselves in a dialogical context where their claims cannot be clearly expressed without risk of misunderstanding or devaluation.

This risk, however, cannot be avoided once and for all. It is not possible to foresee how an agent will interpret their culture, how their experiences will interact with their values and reasons, what values they will embrace and how these values will be shaped by the context. For all these reasons, there is no dialogical model that guarantees the absence of any kind of oppression. Nevertheless, it is possible to radically lower this risk by doing four things:

1. *Paying attention to the effective dialogical answerability and transparency exercised by the medico-juridical assessors.* Assessors must remain open to the possibility that the patient's claims challenge or conflict with their own values and assumptions. In such cases, they should articulate and critically reflect on their starting points, reformulating their reasoning in light of what emerges through the dialogue.

2. *Recognizing the patient's claims, reasons and values, especially in those cases in which these factors could imply the subversion, reformulation or negotiation of current norms and of the values endorsed by the medico-juridical framework.* This task is best undertaken by a multidisciplinary team (e.g. doctors, psychologists, psychiatrists, judges, bioethicists, social workers, carers), whose varied perspectives can balance implicit biases and reduce the risk of oppressive interpretations. The assessment should be the result of democratic deliberation: if one assessor misjudges the patient's dialogical answerability or brings in problematic assumptions, others can moderate or correct these influences.
3. *Taking account of the role and claims of the patient's family, friends, health carers and significant others, and allowing their direct participation in the process of assessment.* These relations are not only deeply affected by the patient's decisions but also provide privileged, historically grounded insights into the patient's values and identity. Their involvement helps create a context conducive to dialogue and reflects the fact that anorexic patients rarely arrive at a non-egosyntonic understanding of their condition in isolation. Supportive relationships are often crucial not only to recognize anorexia as a mental disorder rather than a lifestyle or authentic self-expression but also in overcoming the disorder itself.
4. *Taking account of the dynamics of power involved in the relation between patient and medical establishment.* As Foucault noted,[41] medical discourse is historically entangled with structures of power and knowledge.[42] In the case of anorexia – where most patients are women – gendered power dynamics can distort the assessment process.[43] While no single solution can fully eliminate this risk, some steps can mitigate it. In the short term, anti-oppression and inclusion training tailored to the case at hand could be offered to assessors.[44] Given the urgency of many cases, this may not always be feasible. A more sustainable and far-reaching measure would involve incorporating critical studies of oppression, privilege and power into the academic training of relevant professionals. Given the inherently dialogical and social nature of their work, such education would have lasting value beyond the assessment context.

If the patient fails the initial dialogical answerability assessment, further sessions should be arranged, focusing specifically on observing the conditions outlined earlier. Assessors must gather as much information as possible about the patient's values, reasons, claims and self-regarding attitudes and be ready to express their own values transparently, without assuming their superiority. Given the likely disagreements between assessors and anorexic patients, it is essential 'to take into consideration other, often extra-legal factors – the condition of care, the individual's self-conception, the specific relational context, the type of knowledge one thinks is relevant – or the hypergoods that move us – the primary values of life, the priority of individual choice, the importance of human dignity, the good of social inclusion'.[45]

If, for instance, the dialogue concerns the value of self-control, assessors must consider the patient's understanding of it, without trying to impose a different one. Assessors can appeal to what the patient already accepts, to what she considers important, relevant or valuable. Following Charles Taylor's *ad hominem* approach to moral disputes,[46] the aim isn't to persuade the patient to adopt new principles but to work within their own value framework. With this in mind, assessors would explore in dialogue with the patient the viability of the possible course of action proposed.

As Serene Khader writes, 'What is important for autonomy is knowing what one values and choosing the option on the menu that is most consistent with it.'[47] If, for instance, the patient affirms that 'self-starving guarantees self-control', but also that 'she does not want to die or to harm her family', the assessors could ask her why she actually privileges the former value against the latter. Since the link between self-starving and self-control is a symptom of a treatable condition, assessors can argue that self-control can be achieved in healthier, non-maladaptive ways. In doing so, the patient's values – self-control, care for loved ones, survival – can be aligned.

However, moving towards this sustainable form of self-control requires certain preconditions: weight restoration, letting go of egosyntonic identity traits and building self-worth and self-trust. These are achievable but challenging, especially for those with egosyntonic symptoms or fear of weight gain. Faced with this, how might a patient respond? And how should her dialogical answerability be evaluated? Let us consider these questions.

Take the hypothetical case of a patient who has never received treatment – I'll examine severe and enduring anorexia in the next section – who passes the functional mental capacity test but refuses life-saving treatment. They say that anorexia gives them self-control, yet they also insist they do not want to die or harm their family. In response to the assessors' reflections on possible options, how might they reply? Many replies are possible, depending on the specific case. Still, we can consider some likely examples:

a) The patient might affirm that even if a part of them thinks treatment is the best option, she is unable to consent to it, and she does not deserve it.

In this case, the patient demonstrates a lack of self-worth or self-trust. The forms of self-trust or self-worth they do hold are egosyntonic and fail to address her deeper concerns. Though better alternatives exist – by their own standards – they either see themselves as incapable of pursuing them or unworthy of doing so. For this reason, they cannot be considered capable of deciding on life-saving treatment. As argued in Chapter 5, both self-trust and, above all, self-worth are necessary conditions for the exercise of autonomy.

b) The patient might affirm that they are too much scared of food and of gaining weight to consent to treatment.

If assessors must appeal to what the patient values, they cannot label this fear as irrational – since, from the patient's perspective, fear of food is tied to the value they place on thinness and self-control. Judging this fear as irrational would mean assuming their values and goals are irrational. Moreover, any argument that treats this fear as a symptom explained by the diagnosis of anorexia is flawed. As Giordano notes, 'However common, all of these claims are empty, tautological claims. They involve taking the description for an explanation … Anorexia cannot be the cause (efficient cause) of anything, because we do not know what anorexia is – it is only a name given to a cluster of familiar experience and behaviours.'[48]

A patient who fears food may still want to live, avoid harming loved ones and develop sustainable forms of self-worth and self-trust. Their fear does not block capacity due to irrationality but because it undermines self-trust in their capacity to undertake treatment. Specifically, the patient lacks self-trust about the exercise of their autonomy: they may recognize treatment as the best option but see themselves as unable to act on it due to overwhelming fear. At this point, the patient may even admit that treatment is necessary – but also say they cannot undertake it. Therefore, they should be considered unable to refuse treatment.

c) The patient might admit they need help to undertake and complete treatment.

Here, the patient has reached a clearer understanding of their condition: they recognize the role of others, see anorexia as a problem and accept it as a mental disorder. To reach this point, assessors must avoid imposing their views or trying to persuade them to adopt unfamiliar principles. Instead, they should show how, based on their own values and reasons, better options than refusing treatment are available.

This patient is open to treatment but struggles to maintain that decision. Their attitude may waver – especially during the first stages of treatment – which is precisely when support from caregivers and loved ones becomes most vital. Ongoing and well-calibrated relational support can play a key role in helping her stay aligned with their non-anorexic goals.

d) The patient might affirm that only anorexia can offer the kind of self-control they need.

This case is more complex. Assessors can respond that the patient has no solid reason to be *sure* that *only* anorexia can offer the kind of self-control they need – especially if they've never explored or transitioned to non-anorexic forms of self-control. Since anorexia's symptoms can often be overcome and around 50 per cent of treated patients fully recover,[49] there's no strong basis for rejecting treatment or dismissing the possibility of achieving self-control through healthier means.

How might the patient reject this argument? Perhaps by insisting that *anorexic self-control is unique and cannot be compared to ordinary forms.* Assessors could then ask whether this anorexic self-control is seen as a 'superior' good – one that renders all other values, like health or relationships, trivial or irrelevant.[50] Given the patient's stance, it's likely they would confirm this view, placing anorexic self-control above all else.[51]

> We [anorexics] are 'thrivers'! We thrive upon challenge, upon competition, upon the raw stimulation of life, keenness of our senses, strength and artistry in our bodies, alertness and clarity in our minds. We thrive upon the fact that while all religions, philosophies, ideologies upon the earth extol the virtues of self-control and self-government, our path alone holds the key to unlock the most secret chambers of these mysteries in something so seemingly simple as an empty plate, in something so seemingly shallow as a desire to be thin.[52]

How might the patient respond to the question: *what makes anorexic self-control a 'superior' form of self-control? How does it work?* There are, of course, many possible replies, but two stand out.

First, the patient might claim that *only people with anorexia truly understand anorexic self-control.* In response, assessors could ask why many people with anorexia in treatment and post-anorexics describe that self-control as illusory and oppressive. The patient might dismiss these views, arguing that those who abandon anorexia are no 'real' anorexics, and thus their accounts lack legitimacy.[53] This position is deeply problematic from a dialogical standpoint: the patient appears closed off to any critique that challenges their view. Anorexic self-control is treated as unquestionable, accessible only to those who 'embody' anorexia. In such a scenario, it's unclear whether the patient truly reflects on this value or is simply under the influence of anorexia in a way that bypasses her reflective agency. By rejecting alternative perspectives – including those of other people with anorexia – the patient shows an inability to critically examine the paramount value they place on anorexic self-control. As a result, they cannot be considered able to refuse life-saving treatment.

Second, the patient might say that *anorexic self-control guarantees dominion over one's life, that it makes them feel powerful and safe.* Again, assessors can question why many anorexics and post-anorexics describe this control as ultimately deceptive and oppressive. They might also ask how this control functions in relation to other life domains – such as relationships.[54] If anorexic self-control offers true mastery, why does it conflict with other values the patient themselves hold? Why does it seem, even by her own standards, *less* fulfilling? Moreover, based on their own descriptions, it's unclear why *only* anorexia can guarantee control and safety, or what makes this form of control fundamentally incompatible with other, 'more trivial', forms of self-control.

Even in this case, the patient does not critically engage with alternative views or offer reflective reasons for her certainty. Their belief in the superiority of anorexic control is not the result of a reflective process and fails to account for conflicting data. Given their reasons, the available evidence, the possible outcomes and the irreversible nature of refusing life-saving treatment, there are strong grounds to doubt the validity of their conviction. Thus, they fail to meet the criteria of dialogical answerability and cannot be considered capable of refusing treatment.

e) The patient might affirm that the assessors are missing some relevant issue, that their reasons and values have not been properly taken into account.

In this case, it's crucial not only to understand whether and why the patient feels alienated or oppressed by the dialogical setting but also to create conditions that allow them to clearly express their concerns. They might only be able to articulate their values in familiar environments or with the support of certain significant others. If so, it may be necessary to involve these people in the assessment, taking their input seriously and including them in the dialogue.

Still, the patient may also feel estranged or even oppressed by family or friends, and their involvement could exacerbate their reaction. In such cases, assessors should ask which values or reasons the patient feels are being ignored, or why they don't feel 'safe' enough to articulate them. They might then share more about the values guiding their choices or the kind of oppression they feel in this context. The assessors would need to adjust their arguments accordingly, adopting a dialogical stance that reflects these concerns.

Yet, again, the patient might offer arguments similar to those discussed in the previous case: that only 'real' anorexics can understand their values, that true recognition of anorexic self-control requires accepting it as a supreme good, or that the only way to respect them is to allow refusal of treatment. They might claim the oppression they feel is tied to the assessors' inability to recognize them as a *willing* person with anorexia. For the same reasons discussed earlier, such a stance fails the test of dialogical answerability. The patient cannot be considered capable of refusing treatment.

While no universal model for assessing dialogical answerability can be offered, it's important to note that, in this framework, the patient will likely undergo medical treatment – whether willingly or not. In most cases, a non-egosyntonic, negative view of anorexia only emerges *after* treatment and with the support of others. Looking back, both post-anorexics and those in treatment often acknowledge that some of their earlier choices were not autonomous, and that intervention was ultimately necessary.

Participant 21: I found in the end that if I had wanted to make any choice, different choices that I couldn't do it so it wasn't, it wasn't really my own choice any more.[55]

Participant 18: If [anorexia] almost does become part of you and so in order to get it out of you I think you do have to kind of hurt you in the process, I think it's almost inevitable.[56]

Participant 20: So I didn't really want treatment, but then there's this little voice deep down inside, which is kind of the complex part, that's saying 'you know you do want treatment really', but then there's this kind of overriding big THING which is just like 'no, you're FAT' (laughs), 'you don't need to put on weight!'[57]

We should not conclude that patients who have never received treatment must always be denied the right to refuse life-saving care. Even if, based on dialogical answerability, these patients are found unable to refuse treatment, the reasons why refusal goes against their best interests will still depend on their relational context, personal history, values and concerns. But these relational and personal dimensions matter for another reason: coercive treatment can be especially harmful for patients with anorexia, worsening their sense of lost control and intensifying symptoms. One study shows that compulsory interventions can reduce a patient's ability to engage in psychological therapy;[58] another links forced treatment to higher mortality rates among anorexic patients.[59] Given these risks, it's essential to engage patients in a dialogical process where treatment decisions are explained in relation to their specific concerns. Even if they reject these reasons, they are not treated against their will *because they have anorexia*, but because they cannot exercise autonomy within a relational framework. Their decisional capacity will have been recognized insofar as it has been exercised.

Now let us turn to the case of a patient with severe and enduring anorexia who refuses treatment. First, one clarification: sometimes there is no time for a full assessment of dialogical answerability. In such urgent cases, I believe that untreated anorexic patients should be saved, including through force-feeding if necessary. If the patient is at risk of death, assessment should be postponed until their life is no longer in danger. As I will explain, early intervention greatly improves the chances of recovery – and, as already noted, patients often come to see anorexia as a mental disorder only after receiving care and support.

Refusal of treatment, treatment failures and severe and enduring anorexia

In the literature on eating disorders, the term *severe and enduring* refers to patients who are resistant to treatment and have lived with the disorder for many years.[60] The DSM-V links anorexia's 'severity' to body mass index,[61] while the National Service Framework for Mental Health notes that 'people with recurrent or severe and enduring mental illness … have complex needs which may require the continuing care of specialist mental health services working effectively with other agencies'.[62] Paul Robinson offers a symptom-based definition: a patient has severe and enduring anorexia when symptoms significantly impair quality of life.[63]

Clinicians typically use 'enduring' to describe cases lasting several years – often more than seven[64] – with repeated failed treatments. However, definitions vary, and researchers stress the need for clearer criteria and more research on this phase of the disorder.[65] In what follows, I will use a broad definition of *severe and enduring anorexia* (SEAN) to refer to patients who have been resistant to treatment, previously treated compulsorily and have had anorexia for over ten years.

Let's consider a patient with SEAN who refuses life-saving treatment. Unlike patients who have never received care, they may have stronger, more grounded reasons to believe treatment is no longer in their best interest. Given their medical history, it's reasonable to assume that previously unsuccessful treatments are unlikely to succeed again.[66] Statistics show that around 20 per cent of anorexic patients never recover, and 20 per cent of anorexia-related deaths are due to suicide.[67] Life can become unbearable for SEAN patients, and the alarming suicide rate clearly reflects this. A patient worn down by years of struggle may say *they are too tired to continue living a life whose quality has become too low.*

What can assessors say in response? Scholars like Robinson, Cave and Tan[68] point out that 'one of the most remarkable aspects of treating eating disorders is that patients do, against all predictions, sometimes recover after 8, 10 and even 20 years of illness'.[69] June Alexander, writer and activist who lived with anorexia for over twenty years, insists that recovery is possible, but only by 'listening more deeply to the patient … [and] sharing stories of illness and recovery'.[70] On the other hand, some researchers argue that, based on current data, 'most patients with SEAN are unlikely to fully recover'.[71] Moreover, it has been observed that recovery rates drop sharply with time, especially after three years.[72] In recent years, Deep Brain Stimulation[73] (DBS) has been explored as a possible treatment for SEAN.[74] While promising, the results are preliminary, and more research is needed to determine if, and to what extent, DBS can constitute a potentially successful form of treatment for SEAN.

What level of success makes refusing treatment unreasonable? What counts as success – 'chance of survival after a further course of feeding? Improved quality of life? Recovery from the eating disorder?'[75] All of these? There's no universal threshold. Each case must be evaluated individually, considering context, personal history and values. At the same time, it's important to recognize that treatment itself can pose fatal risks. Anorexia severely weakens the body, and for some SEAN patients, force-feeding may be dangerous enough to outweigh any potential benefit. In such cases, the risks involved in the treatment simply outweigh the possible benefits, and it appears completely unreasonable to compulsorily treat these patients. While SEAN is not technically a chronic or terminal illness, in some cases the chance of recovery is so slim that it borders on zero.[76] When there's no realistic prospect of recovery or survival, assessors cannot reasonably claim that treatment is in the patient's best interest, even by her own standards.

What about cases where treatment does *not* carry a risk of death? As we've seen, current treatments for anorexia make recovery highly unlikely for SEAN patients. So, assessors can't argue that the patient simply doesn't know treatment won't work – their personal and medical history suggest otherwise. Assessors might instead stress that refusing treatment means not just rejecting a cure but choosing a path that likely leads to death. Yet patients with SEAN are often fully aware of this.[77] Their quality of life can become so diminished that death may seem like a relief. As Giordano points out, however, 'anorexia is not a suicidal choice – many anorexics do not want to die; they do not know how else to live'.[78]

SEAN patients face very limited options. Treatments don't work for them, and life becomes an unbearable burden. In some cases, even friends and family might agree that treatment is no longer the best path. It's understandable – if difficult to accept – that in certain situations life can be overwhelming. Still, it's important to remember that research on SEAN is in its early stages,[79] and treatments for anorexia have improved in recent years.[80] It's not unreasonable to believe that better therapies may emerge in the near future.[81] Moreover, as noted earlier, despite the key role of self-regarding attitudes in recovery, there remains a lack of research on how self-worth, self-respect and self-esteem affect treatment outcomes.[82]

Given the many variables involved, assessing the dialogical answerability of a SEAN patient is far more complex than in the previous cases. On the one hand, a patient 'who has struggled with anorexia for a long time, who … has been already treated compulsorily, may have greater insight into her quality of life and greater capacity to refuse medical treatment than someone who has a shorter history of eating disorders'.[83] Their reasons for refusal, while difficult to accept, may be understandable in light of her history, values and concerns. On the other hand, SEAN is not a terminal illness. Some patients recover even after twenty years. Treatments may improve, particularly if relational autonomy is acknowledged and addressed.[84] And the patient's refusal could still stem from impaired self-worth, self-respect or self-esteem.

Still, I don't believe these considerations are enough to override a well-articulated decision to refuse treatment. As we've seen, autonomy depends on self-regarding attitudes like self-worth, respect and trust. Yet little is known about how these attitudes affect decisional capacity in anorexia, or how they influence recovery. Because of this gap, these dimensions must be evaluated individually in each case during the assessment of dialogical answerability. Importantly, a deeper understanding of their role could help improve both treatment and outcomes for SEAN patients.

I have focused on two opposite cases: anorexic patients who have never received treatment and patients with severe and enduring anorexia (SEAN) who are resistant to typical treatments. Given the complexity of these situations, I must emphasize the importance of *early intervention* and the need to take into account the idea that *intervention should not be limited to those cases in which the life of the patient is in danger*. Researchers agree that early intervention greatly reduces the risk of failure and improves the chances of a positive outcome.[85] Moreover, when treatment begins before a life-threatening stage, it typically avoids force-feeding and is far less distressing for patients. The earlier the diagnosis and intervention, the better the chances of recovery. Further research is needed to develop reliable methods for early detection and to explore how early intervention can be ethically implemented.

By combining the dialogical conception of autonomy developed in the Chapter 5 with weak substantivism, I've been able to both consider anorexic patients' claims and address the normative gap they face. Contrary to what defenders of value-neutrality and proceduralism suggest, it is possible to take into account reasons and values when assessing autonomy without prescribing them. Moral language and dialogical exchange are not just features of autonomy – they are essential to evaluating whether, and to what extent, a person's decisional capacity is impaired. This, as we have seen, is especially relevant in the case of anorexic patients refusing life-saving treatment.

Conclusion

The dialogical constitution of autonomy

I have proposed a conception of autonomy that addresses the ethical, practical and theoretical challenges of evaluating the mental capacity of anorexic patients who refuse life-saving treatment. This conception is logically consistent and suitable for practical and legal application. Through examining liberal and relational notions of autonomy, I concluded that autonomy cannot rely on an isolated, private conception of self-knowledge, as this would lead to theoretical issues, ethical shortcomings and insensitivity towards complex social phenomena. Drawing on Wittgenstein and Taylor, I argue that autonomy and self-knowledge are fundamentally relational and dialogical.

Practically, this implies that having supposedly private reasons, values or motivations – accessible only to oneself – is not sufficient to ensure a person's decisional capacity.[1] It also implies that any workable conception of autonomy must consider the dialogical contexts in which autonomy is actually expressed, articulated and negotiated.

Recent feminist philosophers typically criticize liberal, individualistic views of autonomy.[2] The theories grouped under 'relational autonomy' represent one of the latest efforts to redefine autonomy, aiming to reduce its oppressive elements and increase sensitivity to human vulnerability and interdependence. My approach aligns with these broader efforts, recognizing that human beings are inherently relational and interdependent.

Decisions, dilemmas and responsibility: Inescapable value-ladenness

Central to liberal notions of autonomy is an internalist view of reasons, linked to the idea that autonomy must remain normatively neutral. According to this view, only reasons and values *accepted* by the individual – no matter how irrational, unwise or absent – can be considered when evaluating mental capacity. Thus, autonomous actions derive from internal reasons such as desires, motivations or needs, conceived as private and accessible only by the agent. Consequently, the assessment of decision-making focuses solely on the procedure employed, disregarding the content of the decision itself.

The phenomenon of anorexic patients who refuse treatment reveals significant issues with this internalist approach. Neither internalism nor externalism proves adequate, and my analysis shows that autonomy cannot rest on a purely value-neutral, internalist basis. As Meyers suggests, every theory inherently carries normative commitments, whether explicitly acknowledged or not. There is no fully detached stance towards values, reasons or the supposedly private domain of the self. Any perspective inevitably relies on a normative background that highlights what is valuable in contrast with what is not. Thus, adequately addressing anorexic patients' refusal of treatment requires rethinking autonomy beyond liberal conceptions of value-neutrality and epistemological independence.

Dialogical conditions and exercise of autonomy

As argued, the monological approach seems attractive because it appears *self-evident*. It feels natural to assume that *only I truly know my thoughts, reasons, and motivations*. Yet, this perspective cannot explain what it means to misunderstand one's own mental states. If mental content is exclusively private, individuals become helpless when faced with their own misunderstandings. The refusal of treatment by anorexic patients and the problematic contrast between the MCA and Giordano's solutions highlight this limitation. A strictly monological view would require allowing anorexic patients to refuse treatment, which contradicts psychiatric data, testimonies of people with anorexia and post-anorexics, and empirical evidence. Therefore, the idea of epistemological independence must be rejected and replaced by a relational conception of knowledge.

I have identified four relational conditions – three related to self-regarding attitudes and one to dialogical abilities[3] – which shape this conception of autonomy:

1. Self-worth: Autonomous agents see themselves as worthy of making decisions about their lives and defending or expressing their values and reasons.
2. Self-respect: Autonomous agents adopt a self-caring attitude, accepting their fallibility, vulnerability and interdependence, while rejecting both self-neglect and extreme forms of self-acceptance or self-obsession.
3. Self-trust: Autonomous agents trust their capacity to act according to their reasons and values, trust their ability to act upon these reasons and trust their own judgements.
4. Dialogical accountability: Autonomous agents can engage in meaningful dialogue, articulate, defend and revise their reasons and values through interactions with others.

These four conditions have moral grounding. However, contrary to monological interpretations, they are neither paternalistic nor value-biased, and they do not prescribe or anticipate specific decisions. Instead, they ensure decisions are genuinely autonomous, in the nuanced sense proposed here. By recognizing vulnerability, relational embeddedness and interdependence as inherent human characteristics, this conception also provides a basis for understanding *intervention* not as a justified yet inherently coercive act – typical of monological perspectives – but rather as a practice of *relational responsibility* aimed not only at protecting but also at *enhancing* autonomy.

Future directions

Further research is needed to explore in greater detail the roles played by self-worth, self-respect and self-trust in anorexic and SEAN patients. Although scholars have extensively studied self-esteem (a broader concept overlapping to varying degrees with the attitudes mentioned), the specific contributions of self-worth, self-respect and self-trust remain under-investigated.[4] Given this gap, assessments of these self-regarding attitudes should, for now, be approached carefully, evaluating each patient individually during dialogues assessing answerability. Importantly, a deeper understanding of how these attitudes function in anorexia and SEAN could significantly enhance therapeutic approaches aimed at developing or restoring them.

The dialogical account of agency developed here has drawn on insights provided by anorexic patients and critiques of the autonomy concept within the MCA, particularly concerning treatment refusal. However, this dialogical framework could also be fruitfully applied to other cases involving nuanced treatment refusals, such as those concerning eating disorders more broadly, depression, schizophrenia, dementia and Alzheimer's disease. Examining these cases through a dialogical lens may enrich and expand our understanding of human agency. Moreover, this relational-dialogical approach has implications beyond treatment refusal, including in multiculturalism, pluralism, decolonialism and postcolonialism – in short, wherever human perspectives clash or efforts to establish common ground are crucial.

Glossary

Psychological and medico-legal terms

Adaptive Preferences: Preferences and values shaped by oppressive or limiting conditions. Individuals may internalize diminished expectations, resulting in desires that are responses to their constrained circumstances rather than authentic reflections of their identity.

Asceticism: The deliberate practice of self-denial or strict discipline, often for spiritual or moral purposes.

Best Interests: A medico-legal criterion guiding decisions for individuals lacking decisional capacity. It involves assessing medical, emotional, psychological and social factors to determine the most beneficial outcome for the patient.

Body Dysmorphic Disorder: A psychological condition characterized by obsessive preoccupation with perceived defects or flaws in physical appearance, often trivial or non-existent to others

Body Mass Index (BMI): A numerical measure calculated from a person's height and weight, commonly used to classify underweight, healthy weight, overweight or obesity.

Compensatory Practices: Behaviours aimed at counteracting perceived excessive eating or weight gain. Common compensatory practices include self-induced vomiting, excessive exercise and misuse of laxatives or diuretics.

Compulsive Behaviours: Repetitive, ritualistic actions driven by an intense urge or perceived necessity, often enacted despite adverse consequences.

Court of Protection: A specialized court in England and Wales responsible for decisions involving individuals who lack mental capacity, especially concerning healthcare, welfare and financial matters. It ensures decisions align with the individual's best interests.

Deep Brain Stimulation (DBS): A medical procedure involving the surgical implantation of electrodes in specific brain areas, delivering electrical impulses to regulate abnormal brain activity.

Decisional Capacity: The ability to understand, appreciate, reason about and communicate a decision. Decisional capacity is context-specific, assessed with respect to particular choices.

Delusional Beliefs: Firmly held beliefs maintained despite clear evidence to the contrary, often irrational or unrealistic.

Egosyntony: A psychological state wherein behaviours, values and symptoms are experienced as congruent or consistent with one's self-image and identity.

Functional Test: A medico-legal assessment used to determine mental capacity, typically involving the individual's ability to understand, retain, weigh relevant information and communicate decisions clearly.

Internalized Oppression: The internal acceptance and reinforcement of negative stereotypes or discriminatory beliefs about oneself, often resulting from prolonged exposure to oppressive social contexts.

Intervention: Actions undertaken to support or protect an individual's autonomy and well-being, especially in cases of impaired decisional capacity.

Maladaptive Habits: Learned behavioural patterns that negatively impact an individual's well-being or adaptive functioning.

Mental Capacity: The cognitive ability to make informed and autonomous decisions. In medico-legal contexts, mental capacity is typically evaluated concerning specific decisions.

Motivational Set: The collection of an individual's internal reasons, desires, values and beliefs that inform their decisions and actions.

Reflective Endorsement: The conscious affirmation and acceptance of one's motivations, values and actions upon reflective examination.

Self-Regarding Attitudes: Attitudes that individuals hold about themselves, critically affecting autonomy. Key self-regarding attitudes include self-worth, self-respect and self-trust.

Treatment Refusal: The decision by a patient to decline recommended medical interventions, including life-saving measures.

Philosophical terms

Asymptote: Metaphorically, an ideal or concept approached but never fully attained.

Atomistic Individualism: A view of individuals as entirely self-contained, independent agents, largely unaffected by social and relational contexts.

Authoritarianism: A stance or practice characterized by enforcing strict obedience at the expense of personal autonomy and dialogue.

Causal Relationality: The view that relationships and social contexts causally affect the development of autonomy without fundamentally defining it.

Constitutive Relationality: The understanding that relationships and social contexts fundamentally constitute and define autonomy itself.

Dialogical Accountability: The requirement for autonomous agents to articulate, defend and revise their reasons and values through dialogue with others.

Dialogical Agent: An individual who understands and defines their identity, values and autonomy through interaction and dialogue with others.

Dialogical Constitution: The formation and ongoing shaping of autonomy and identity through relational and dialogical interactions.

Epistemological Independence: The assumption that individuals have private, direct and infallible knowledge of their mental states and motivations, independent of relational contexts.

Externalism of Reasons: The philosophical position that reasons for actions are determined independently of the individual's subjective motivations or desires.

Gender Norms: Socially constructed expectations and standards related to gender roles and behaviours.

Gendered Structures: Institutional and societal arrangements reinforcing gender roles and expectations.
Global Autonomy: The overall capacity of an individual to govern themselves reflectively and authentically throughout significant portions of life.
Heteronomy: A condition of being governed by external forces or influences, as opposed to autonomy.
Instrumental Rationality: A conception of rationality focused solely on efficiency in achieving predetermined goals, irrespective of moral or relational considerations.
Intersectionality: A framework for understanding how multiple social identities intersect and create unique modes of discrimination and privilege.
Internalism of Reasons: The philosophical stance that reasons for action are fundamentally linked to an individual's subjective motivations or desires.
Interdependence: The condition of mutual dependence and influence among individuals.
Local Autonomy: Autonomy concerning specific, context-dependent decisions or actions.
Monological Agent: Atomistic individual perceived as epistemologically independent.
Moral Subjectivism: The view that moral truths and values are based solely on individual preferences or subjective states.
Oppression: Systemic and pervasive forms of discrimination or injustice limiting and defining individuals' autonomy and opportunities.
Ostensive Definition: Defining concepts by directly pointing to examples or instances.
Paternalism: Intervention justified by the claim that it protects or enhances an individual's welfare.
Private Language: The theoretical concept of a language understandable only to its user.
Procedural Autonomy: Autonomy evaluated solely through decision-making processes without considering the content of decisions.
Responsibility: The ethical obligation to account for one's actions and decisions.
Social Embeddedness: The concept that individuals are inherently situated within social contexts shaping their identities, values and autonomy.
Strong Substantivism: The view that autonomy necessarily involves adherence to specific values considered universally valid.
Substantive Autonomy: Autonomy assessed through content-based evaluation of individuals' values and reasons rather than procedural criteria alone.
Value-ladenness: The condition of a theory being grounded in specific values, whether implicitly or explicitly. On this view, normative commitments are integral part of any theory.
Value-neutrality: The claim that a theory can be constructed independently from values or motives.
Value-saturated: A position claiming that only choices and actions following moral or 'right' reasons can be truly considered autonomous. These theories explicitly restrict autonomy to outcomes compatible with a predefined moral framework.
Weak Substantivism: A theory that does not exclude choices based on their moral content but requires the presence of certain capacities – like self-respect or dialogical answerability – as conditions for autonomy.

Notes

Introduction

1 Pamela K. Keel and Tiffany A Brown, 'Update on Course and Outcome in Eating Disorders', *International Journal of Eating Disorders* 43, no. 3 (2010): 195–204.

2 Jon Arcelus, Alex J. Mitchell, Jackie Wales and Søren Nielsen, 'Mortality Rates in Patients with Anorexia Nervosa and Other Eating Disorders: A Meta-Analysis of 36 Studies', *Archives of General Psychiatry* 68, no. 7 (2011): 724–31; Frédérique Smink, Daphne van Hoeken, and Hans W. Hoek, 'Epidemiology of Eating Disorders: Incidence, Prevalence and Mortality Rates', *Current Psychiatry Reports* 14, no. 4 (2012): 406–14; Keel and Brown, 'Update on Course and Outcome in Eating Disorders', 195–204; Arthur Crisp, 'Death, Survival and Recovery in Anorexia Nervosa: A Thirty-Five Year Study', *European Eating Disorders Review* 14, no. 3 (2006): 168–75.

3 Nathalie T. Burkert, *Psychological and Neurobiological Aspects of Eating Disorders: A Taste fMRI Study in Patients Suffering from Anorexia Nervosa* (New York: Springer, 2016), 34.

4 Gareth S. Owen, Fabian Freyenhagen, Genevra Richardson and Matthew Hotopf, 'Mental Capacity and Decisional Autonomy: An Interdisciplinary Challenge', *Inquiry* 52, no. 1 (2009): 79–107.

5 *Re T (Adult: Refusal of Medical Treatment)* (1992) 4 All ER 649 at 669.

6 Simona Giordano, *Understanding Eating Disorders. Conceptual and Ethical Issues in the Treatment of Anorexia and Bulimia Nervosa* (Oxford: Oxford University Press, 2005).

7 Giordano, *Understanding Eating Disorders*; Simona Giordano, 'Anorexia Nervosa and Its Moral Foundations', *International Journal of Children's Rights* 13, nos. 1–2 (2005): 149–60; Simona Giordano, 'Anorexia Nervosa: A Case for Exceptionalism in Ethical Decision Making', *Philosophy, Psychiatry & Psychology* 26, no. 4 (2019): 315–31.

8 In her later work, Giordano moves away from her 'brave claim' and adopts a position closer to that which I propose in this book. I analyse her last proposal in chapter 6. Giordano, 'Anorexia Nervosa'.

9

> This is what I call the brave claim: people with anorexia nervosa who competently decide not to be artificially fed should be respected because everybody is entitled

> to the exercise of their autonomy, not only 'in the middle' of their life, but also at the end of it, or when their own life is at stake. The principle of autonomy binds us to respect people's competent decisions about their life and its termination, precisely because autonomy extends also to the most difficult moments of our life, and, ultimately, 'stretches far out into the distance', to the end of it. (Giordano, *Understanding Eating Disorders*, 246)

10 I am referring in particular to cases of severe and enduring anorexia. The last section of this book is dedicated to this topic.

11 Catriona Mackenzie and Natalie Stoljar, eds, *Relational Autonomy: Feminist Perspectives on Autonomy, Agency, and the Social Self* (Oxford: Oxford University Press, 2000).

12 Mackenzie and Stoljar, *Relational Autonomy.*

13 At a very basic level, all relational scholars think that oppressive social contexts can impair autonomy, but there is no agreement on the conditions governing this possibility. Furthermore, scholars agree that human agents are vulnerable, dependent on others and reliant on the practical availability of goods and opportunities, but they diverge about the details of a notion of the human agent characterized by these characteristics.

14 Paul Benson, 'Free Agent and Self-Worth', *Journal of Philosophy* 91, no. 12 (1994): 656–7.

15 I consider self-esteem a subcategory or a synonym of self-worth. This topic will be further explored in Chapters 4 and 5.

16 Self-worth is a necessary condition not only for the exercise of autonomy but also for the development and sustainment of other self-regarding attitudes connected to autonomy, such as *self-respect* and *self-trust*. Both these self-regarding attitudes overlap in many ways with self-worth, but they have their specific focus on other aspects of the agent's self-consideration. In the fourth, sixth and especially fifth chapters, I analyse in depth the relations between self-worth, self-esteem, self-respect and self-trust.

17 Catriona Mackenzie, 'Three Dimension of Autonomy: A Relational Analysis', in *Autonomy, Oppression, and Gender*, ed. Andrea Veltman and Mark Piper (Oxford: Oxford University Press, 2014), 38.

Chapter 1

1 World Health Organization, *The ICD-10 Classification of Mental and Behavioural Disorders: Clinical Descriptions and Diagnostic Guidelines* (Geneva: World Health Organization, 1992); American Psychiatric Association, *Diagnostic and Statistical Manual of Mental Disorders*, 5th edn (Arlington, VA: American Psychiatric, 2013).

2 Sophie C. Norris, David H. Gleaves and Amanda D. Hutchinson, 'Anorexia Nervosa and Perfectionism: A Meta-Analysis', *International Journal of Eating Disorders* 52, no. 3 (2019): 219–29; Janet Polivy and Peter C. Herman, 'Causes of Eating Disorders', *Annual Review of Psychology* 53 (2002): 187–213; Ellen E. Walters and Kenneth S. Kendler, 'Anorexia Nervosa and Anorexic-Like Syndromes in a Population-Based Female Twin Sample', *American Journal of Psychiatry* 152, no. 1 (1995): 64–71.

3 Giordano, *Understanding Eating Disorders*, 137.

4 Kathleen K. Fitzpatrick and James Lock, 'Anorexia Nervosa', *Psychiatric Clinics of North America* 34, no. 4 (2011): 849–59.

5 Katarina K. Lindstedt, Lars Kjellin and Sanna A. Gustafsson, 'Adolescents with Full or Subthreshold Anorexia Nervosa in a Naturalistic Sample: Characteristics and Treatment Outcome', *Journal of Eating Disorders* 5, no. 4 (2017): 1–13; Stephan Zipfel, Katrin E. Giel, Cynthia M. Bulik, Phillipa Hay and Ulrike Schmidt, 'Anorexia Nervosa: Aetiology, Assessment and Treatment', *Lancet Psychiatry* 2, no. 12 (2015): 1099–111.

6 Sara Kakhi and Jacinta McCann, 'Anorexia Nervosa: Diagnosis, Risk Factors and Evidence-Based Treatments', *Progress in Neurology and Psychiatry* 20, no. 6 (2016): 24–29c.

7 Crisp, 'Death Survival and Recovery'; Burkert, *Psychological and Neurobiological Aspects of Eating Disorders*, 39.

8 Smink, van Hoeken and Hoek, 'Epidemiology of Eating Disorders'.

9 According to some scholars, anorexia is not a disorder strictly connected to Western culture but to cultures in transition to urbanization and globalization. Dattatreya N. Mendhekar, Kavita Arora, Deep Lohia, Ashish Aggarwal and Ram C. Jiloha, 'Anorexia Nervosa: An Indian Perspective', *National Medical Journal of India* 22, no. 4 (2009): 181–2; Mervat Nasser, 'Eating Disorders across Cultures', *Psychiatry* 6, no. 9 (2009): 347–50.

10 An increasing occurrence of anorexia has been found in non-western country such as India, China, Japan, South Africa, Iran, Tanzania and Malaysia; Jane Wardle, Renu Bindra, Beverley Fairclough and Alex Westcombe, 'Culture and Body Image: Body Perception and Weight Concern in Young Asian and Caucasian British Women', *Journal of Community & Applied Social Psychology* 3, no. 3 (1993): 173–81; Aya Nishizono-Maher, 'Eating Disorders in Japan: Finding the Right Context', *Psychiatry and Clinical Neurosciences* 52, suppl. (1998): S320–3; Daniel le Grange, Christy F. Telch and Jason Tibbs, 'Eating Attitudes and Behaviors in 1435 South African Caucasian and Non-Caucasian College Students', *American Journal of Psychiatry* 155, no. 2 (1998): 250–4; Kamryn T. Eddy, Moira Hennessey and Heather Thompson-Brenner, 'Eating Pathology in East African Women: The Role of Media Exposure and Globalization', *Journal of Nervous and Mental Disease* 195, no. 3 (2007): 196–202; Jacinta Tan, Syahirah A. Karim, Huei Y. Lee and Goh L. Yen, 'Cultural and Ethical Issues in the Treatment of Eating Disorders in Singapore', *Asian Bioethics Review* 5, no.

1 (2013): 40–55; Kathleen M. Pike and Patricia E. Dunne, 'The Rise of Eating Disorders in Asia: A Review', *Journal of Eating Disorders* 3, no. 1 (2015): 33.

11 Even if anorexia has been considered a typical feminine disorder, it also affects the male population, but with a lower incidence (0.2–0.3 per cent) and prevalence (4–5 per cent). Stuart B. Murray, Jason M. Nagata, Scott Griffiths, Jerel P. Calzo, Tiffany A. Brown, Deborah Mitchison, Aaron J. Blashill and Jonathan M. Mond, 'The Enigma of Male Eating Disorders: A Critical Review and Synthesis', *Clinical Psychology Review* 57 (2017): 1–11.

12 Antonio Preti, Ambra Usai, Paola Miotto, Donatella Rita Petretto and Carmelo Masala, 'Eating Disorders among Professional Fashion Models', *Psychiatry Research* 159, nos. 1–2 (2008): 86–94; Jon Arcelus, Gemma L. Witcomb and Alex Mitchell, 'Prevalence of Eating Disorders amongst Dancers: A Systematic Review and Meta-Analysis', *European Eating Disorders Review* 22, no. 2 (2014): 92–101.

13 Hans W. Hoek, 'Distribution of Eating Disorders', in *Eating Disorders and Obesity: A Comprehensive Handbook*, ed. Kelly D. Brownell and Cristopher G. Fairburn (New York: Guilford Press, 1995), 233–38.

14 Evelyn Attia, 'Anorexia Nervosa: Current Status and Future Directions', *Annual Review of Medicine* 61 (2010): 425–35.

15 Amélie Kipman, Philip Gorwood, Marie-Christine Mouren-Siméoni and Jacques Adès, 'Genetic Factors in Anorexia Nervosa', *European Psychiatry* 14, no. 4, (1999): 189–98.

16 American Psychiatric Association, *Diagnostic and Statistical Manual*.

17 Giordano, *Understanding Eating Disorders*; Paula Saukko, *The Anorexic Self: A Personal, Political Analysis of a Diagnostic Discourse* (New York: State University of New York Press, 2008); Sigal Gooldin, 'Being Anorexic: Hunger, Subjectivity, and Embodied Morality', *Medical Anthropology Quarterly*. 22, no. 3 (2008): 274–96.

18 John M. S. Pearce, 'Richard Morton: Origins of Anorexia Nervosa', *European Neurology* 52, no. 4 (2004): 191–2.

19 Walter Vandereycken, 'History of Anorexia Nervosa and Bulimia Nervosa', in *Eating Disorders and Obesity: A Comprehensive Handbook*, ed. Kelly D. Brownell and Cristopher G. Fairburn (New York: Guilford Press, 1995): 151–5.

20 Vandereycken, 'History of Anorexia'.

21 Vandereycken, 'History of Anorexia'.

22 Vandereycken, 'History of Anorexia'.

23 Pearce, 'Richard Morton'.

24 Fernando E. Forcen, 'Anorexia Mirabilis: The Practice of Fasting by Saint Catherine of Siena in the Late Middle Ages', *American Journal of Psychiatry* 170, no. 4 (2013): 370–1.

25 Cybelle Weinberg, 'From the Ascetic Ideal to the Esthetic Ideal: The Historical Evolution of Anorexia Nervosa', *Revista Latinoamericana de Psicopatologia Fundamental* 13, no. 2 (2010): 224–37.

26 Pearce, 'Richard Morton'.

27 Anna K. Silver, *Victorian Literature and the Anorexic Body* (Cambridge: Cambridge University Press, 2002); Emma Domínguez-Rué, 'Sins of the Flesh: Anorexia, Eroticism and the Female Vampire in Bram Stoker's Dracula', *Journal of Gender Studies* 19, no. 3 (2010): 297–308.

28 Tony Hope, Jacinta Tan, Anne Stewart and Ray Fitzpatrick, 'Anorexia Nervosa and the Language of Authenticity', *Hastings Center Report* 41, no. 6 (2011): 19–29; Jacinta Tan, Tony Hope and Anne Stewart, 'Anorexia Nervosa and Personal Identity: The Accounts of Patients and Their Parents', *International Journal of Law and Psychiatry* 26, no. 5 (2003): 533–48; Jacinta Tan, Anne Stewart, Raymond Fitzpatrick and Tony Hope, 'Attitudes of Patients with Anorexia Nervosa to Compulsory Treatment and Coercion', *International Journal of Law and Psychiatry* 33, no. 1 (2010): 13–19; Tony Hope, Jacinta Tan, Anne Stewart and John McMillan, 'Agency, Ambivalence and Authenticity: The Many Ways in Which Anorexia Nervosa Can Affect Autonomy', *International Journal of Law in Context* 9, no. 1 (2013): 20–36; Jacinta Tan, Tony Hope, Anne Stewart and Raymond Fitzpatrick, 'Control and Compulsory Treatment in Anorexia Nervosa: The Views of Patients and Parents', *International Journal of Law and Psychiatry* 26, no. 6 (2003): 627–45; Jacinta Tan, Tony Hope, Anne Stewart and Raymond Fitzpatrick, 'Competence to Make Treatment Decisions in Anorexia Nervosa: Thinking Processes and Values', *Philosophy, Psychiatry, & Psychology* 13 (2006): 267–82; Jacinta Tan, Tony Hope and Anne Stewart, 'Competence to Refuse Treatment in Anorexia Nervosa', *International Journal of Law and Psychiatry* 26, no. 6 (2003): 697–707.

29 Tan, Hope and Stewart, 'Anorexia Nervosa and Personal Identity'.

30 Tan, Hope and Stewart, 'Anorexia Nervosa and Personal Identity'.

31 Hope, Tan, Stewart and Fitzpatrick, 'Anorexia Nervosa and the Language of Authenticity'.

32 Tan, Hope and Stewart, 'Anorexia Nervosa and Personal Identity'.

33 Hope, Tan, Stewart and McMillan, 'Agency, Ambivalence and Authenticity'.

34 Hope, Tan, Stewart and Fitzpatrick, 'Anorexia and the Language of Authenticity'.

35 Hope, Tan, Stewart and Fitzpatrick, 'Anorexia and the Language of Authenticity'.

36 Hope, Tan, Stewart and Fitzpatrick, 'Anorexia and the Language of Authenticity'.

37 Hope, Tan, Stewart and Fitzpatrick, 'Anorexia and the Language of Authenticity'.

38 *Special Books by Special Kids*, 'Battling Chronic Anorexia for Over a Decade (But Still Fighting for Recovery)'. YouTube video, 15:55. Posted 2 November 2018. https://www.youtube.com/watch?v=NOoNYdhYOWY.

39 Tan, Hope, Stewart and Fitzpatrick, 'Control and Compulsory Treatment in Anorexia'.

40 *Special Books by Special Kids*, 'Battling Chronic Anorexia'.

41 Leslie R. Shade, 'Weborexics: The Ethical Issues Surrounding Pro-Ana Websites', *ACM SIGCAS Computers and Society* 33, no. 4 (2003): 2.

42 Anna Gwizdek, Katarzyna Gwizdek and Agnieszka Koszowska, 'Pro-Ana, Murderous Face of the Internet', *Progress in Health Sciences* 2, no. 1 (2012): 158–61.

43 Samantha R. Strife and Kathryn Rickard, 'The Conceptualization of Anorexia: The Pro-Ana Perspective', *Affilia* 26, no. 2 (2011): 213–17.

44 Nicole D. Schott and Debra Langan, 'Pro-Anorexia/Bulimia Censorship and Public Service Announcements: The Price of Controlling Women', *Media, Culture & Society* 37, no. 8 (2015): 1158–73.

45 Tan, Hope, Stewart and Fitzpatrick, 'Control and Compulsory Treatment in Anorexia'.

46 Louis C. Charland, Tony Hope, Anne Stewart and Jacinta Tan, 'Anorexia Nervosa as a Passion', *Philosophy, Psychiatry, & Psychology* 20, no. 4 (2013): 353–65.

47 Tan, Hope, Stewart and Fitzpatrick, 'Treatment Decisions in Anorexia Nervosa'.

48 Tan, Hope, Stewart and Fitzpatrick, 'Treatment Decisions in Anorexia Nervosa'.

49 Hope, Tan, Stewart and McMillan, 'Agency, Ambivalence and Authenticity'.

50 Tan, Hope and Stewart, 'Competence to Refuse Treatment in Anorexia'.

51 Louis Theroux, *Louis Theroux: Talking to Anorexia*, documentary, BBC, 2017.

52 Hope, Tan, Stewart and McMillan, 'Agency, Ambivalence and Authenticity'.

53 Hope, Tan, Stewart and McMillan, 'Agency, Ambivalence and Authenticity'.

54 Janet E. Conti, 'Recovering Identity from Anorexia Nervosa: Women's Constructions of Their Experiences of Recovery from Anorexia Nervosa Over 10 Years', *Journal of Constructivist Psychology* 31, no. 1 (2018): 72–94.

55 Hope, Tan, Stewart and Fitzpatrick, 'Anorexia Nervosa and the Language of Authenticity'.

56 Conti, 'Recovering Identity'.

57 Hope, Tan, Stewart and Fitzpatrick, 'Anorexia Nervosa and the Language of Authenticity'.

58 Conti, 'Recovering Identity'.

59 Conti, 'Recovering Identity'.

60 Conti, 'Recovering Identity'.

61 Conti, 'Recovering Identity'.

62 Conti, 'Recovering Identity'; Giordano, *Understanding Eating Disorders*; Saukko, *The Anorexic Self*.

63 Saukko, *The Anorexic Self*, 6.

64 Saukko, *The Anorexic Self*, 9.

65 Saukko, *The Anorexic Self*, 105.

66 Saukko, *The Anorexic Self*, 60.

67 Saukko, *The Anorexic Self*, 82.

68 Schott, 'Pro-Anorexia/Bulimia Censorship'; Gwizdek, 'Murderous Face of the Internet'; Strife, 'The Conceptualization of Anorexia'; Shade, 'Weborexics'.

69 American Psychiatric Association, *Diagnostic and Statistical Manual*; Greg Dring, 'Anorexia Runs in Families: Is This Due to Genes or the Family Environment', *Journal of Family Therapy* 37, no. 1 (2015): 79–92.

70 Mara S. Palazzoli, Stefano Cirillo, Matteo Selvini and Anna M. Sorrentino , *Ragazze Anoressiche e Bulimiche: La Terapia Familiare* (Milano: Cortina, 1998).

71 Anna Goodman, Amy Heshmati and Ilona Koupil, 'Family History of Education Predicts Eating Disorders across Multiple Generations among 2 Million Swedish Males and Females', *PLoS ONE* 9, no. 8 (2014): 1–9.

72 Lisa McClelland and Arthur Crisp, 'Anorexia Nervosa and Social Class', *International Journal of Eating Disorders* 29, no. 2 (2001): 150–6; L. Lindberg and A. Hjern, 'Risk Factors for Anorexia Nervosa: A National Cohort Study', *International Journal of Eating Disorders* 34, no. 4 (2003): 397–408; J. C. Ahrén, Flaminia Chiesa, Ilona Koupil, Cecilia Magnusson, Christina Dalman and Anna Goodman, 'We Are Family – Parents, Siblings, and Eating Disorders in a Prospective Total-Population Study of 250,000 Swedish Males and Females', *International Journal of Eating Disorders* 46, no. 7 (2013): 693–700.

73 The results of this study are valid only in those countries in which education is free and, as a consequence, where the level of income is not crucially related to the level of education.

74 Hilde Bruch, *Eating Disorders: Obesity, Anorexia Nervosa and the Person Within* (London: Routledge and Kegan Paul, 1974), 262; Palazzoli, Cirillo, Selvini and Sorrentino, *Ragazze Anoressiche*, 22–3, 122.

75 Ahrén reads the data in a different way, claiming that anorexia is found more commonly between families with higher level of education since increased knowledge makes the parents more aware of mental disorders and more prompt to ask for medical help. Jennie C. Ahrén, Flaminia Chiesa, Britt A. Klinteberg and Ilona Koupil, 'Psychosocial Determinants and Family Background in Anorexia Nervosa: Results from the Stockholm Birth Cohort Study', *International Journal of Eating Disorders* 45, no. 3 (2012): 362–9; Kathleen M. Pike, Anja Hilbert, Denise E. Wilfley, Christopher G. Fairburn, Faith-Anne Dohm, Bernard T. Walsh and Ruth H. Striegel-Moore, 'Toward an Understanding of Risk Factors for Anorexia Nervosa: A Case-Control Study', *Psychological Medicine* 38, no. 10 (2008): 1443–53; Dring, 'Anorexia Runs in Families',

79–92; Ivan Eisler, Christopher Dare, Matthew Hodes, Gerald F. Russell, Elizabeth Dodge and Daniel le Grange, 'Family Therapy for Adolescent Anorexia Nervosa: The Results of a Controlled Comparison of Two Family Interventions', *Journal of Child Psychology and Psychiatry, and Allied Disciplines* 41, no. 6 (2000): 727–36.

76 Goodman, Heshmati and Koupil, 'Family History of Education Predicts Eating Disorders'.

77 Goodman, Heshmati and Koupil, 'Family History of Education Predicts Eating Disorders'.

78 Palazzoli, Cirillo, Selvini and Sorrentino, *Ragazze Anoressiche*.

79 Interestingly, this argument parallels to the 1960 literature on mental illness and Bateson's account of schizophrenia. Ronald D. Laing and Aaron Esterson, *Sanity, Madness, and the Family* (London: Penguin Books, 1964); Gregory Bateson, *Steps to an Ecology of Mind* (Chicago: University of Chicago Press, 1972), part III.

80 Barton J. Blinder, Edward J. Cumella and Visant A. Sanathara, 'Psychiatric Comorbidities of Female Inpatients with Eating Disorders', *Psychosomatic Medicine* 68, no. 3 (2006): 454–62.

81 Bateson, *Ecology of Mind*, part III.

82 Domínguez-Rué, 'Sins of the Flesh'.

83 Susan Bordo, *Unbearable Weight: Feminism, Western Culture, and the Body* (Berkeley: University of California Press, 1993), 8, 160–1, emphasis in original.

84 Bordo, *Unbearable Weight*, 142.

85 Bordo, *Unbearable Weight*, 155, emphasis in original.

86 I distinguish between 'soft' and 'hard' explicative approaches. A 'hard' explanation claims to have identified the causal elements (x) of a determinate phenomenon (k) (x causes k), while a 'soft' explanation looks at the relation between the variable identified and the phenomenon in terms of probability (k is present at higher rates in presence of x).

87 Saukko, *The Anorexic Self*, 4, 103.

88 Saukko, *The Anorexic Self*, 108.

89 Saukko, *The Anorexic Self*, 108.

90 Saukko, *The Anorexic Self*, 59–76, 80–1, 106–10.

91 Saukko, *The Anorexic Self*, 3, 108.

92 Saukko, *The Anorexic Self*, 164–9.

93 Saukko, *The Anorexic Self*, 169–71.

94 Giordano, *Understanding Eating Disorders*, 158–60, 172.

95 Giordano, 'Anorexia Nervosa and Its Moral Foundations'.

96 Giordano, *Understanding Eating Disorders*, 258.

97 Giordano, *Understanding Eating Disorders*, 262–4.

98 Giordano, *Understanding Eating Disorders*; Hannah Bowden, 'Is Anorexia Nervosa a Passion?', *Philosophy, Psychiatry, & Psychology* 20, no. 4 (2013): 367–70, 381. For the phenomenological priority of the affective dimension from a philosophical, neurobiological and anthropological point of view see respectively: Charles Taylor and Hubert Dreyfus, *Retrieving Realism* (Cambridge, MA: Harvard University Press, 2015); Jaak Panksepp and Lucy Biven, *The Archeology of the Mind: Neuroevolutionary Origins of Human Emotions* (London: W. W. Norton, 2012); Michael Tomasello, *Origins of Human Communication* (Cambridge, MA: MIT Press, 2008).

Chapter 2

1 Department for Constitutional Affairs, *Mental Capacity Act 2005: Code of Practice* (London: TSO, 2007), 48.

2 *Mental Capacity Act 2005* (London: HMSO, 2005) – hereafter referred to as the 'MCA'.

3 *Re T (Adult: Refusal of Medical Treatment)* [1992] EWCA Civ 18.

4 MCA, c. 2.

5 According to the functional test a person's decisional capacity is determined by her understanding of the matter, and not by the content of her outcome. This can be considered a procedural, value-neutral approach to a person's capacities, as opposed to a substantial, value-laden approach.

6 Thomas Grisso, Paul S. Appelbaum and Carolyn Hill-Fotouhi, 'The MacCAT-T: A Clinical Tool to Assess Patients' Capacities to Make Treatment Decisions', *Psychiatric Services* 48, no. 11 (1997): 1415–19.

7 Tan, Hope and Stewart, 'Anorexia Nervosa and Personal Identity'; Tan, Hope, Stewart and Fitzpatrick, 'Control and Compulsory Treatment in Anorexia'; Tan, Hope, Stewart and Fitzpatrick, 'Competence to Make Treatment Decisions in Anorexia'; Tan, Karim, Lee and Yen, 'Cultural and Ethical Issues in the Treatment of Eating Disorders'.

8

> Under a section 2 (s2), you are detained in hospital for assessment of your mental health and to get any treatment you might need … Under a s2 you can't refuse treatment … Under a section 3 (s3), you are detained in hospital for treatment. Treatment might be necessary for your health, your safety or for the protection of other people … Under a s3 you can't refuse treatment. You can be treated against your will. (*Mental Health Act 1983* (London: HMSO, 1983) – hereafter referred to as the 'MHA')

9 *A Local Authority v E* [2012] EWCOP 1639.

10 Wang, 'Mental Capacity Act'.

11 Stephen Touyz, Phillip Aouad, Terry Carney, Shu Hwa Ong, Joel Yager, Richard Newton, Phillipa Hay, Sarah Maguire and Emma Bryant, 'Clinical, Legal and Ethical Implications of Coercion and Compulsory Treatment in Eating Disorders: Do Rapid Review Findings Identify Clear Answers or More Muddy Waters?', *Journal of Eating Disorders* 12, no. 163 (2024): 1–16.

12 Royal College of Psychiatrists and Royal College of Physicians, *MARSIPAN: Management of Really Sick Patients with Anorexia Nervosa*, 2nd edn, College Report CR189 (2014): 51–2.

13 Giordano, *Understanding Eating Disorders*, 179–210.

14 Mental Health Act Commission, *Guidance on the Treatment of Anorexia under the Mental Health Act 1983* (London: HMSO, 1997).

15 Department of Health and Welsh Office, *Code of Practice: Mental Health Act 1983* (London: Stationery Office, 1999).

16 *A NHS Foundation Trust v MS X* [2014] EWCOP 35.

17 *A NHS Foundation Trust v MS X*.

18 Giordano, *Understanding Eating Disorders*, 70.

19 'Why do you manifest the following disturbances? … Because you suffer from anorexia. (tautological answer) = You manifest the following disturbances because you manifest the following disturbances (having anorexia nervosa, in fact, means that you are manifesting the following disturbances)' (Giordano, *Understanding Eating Disorders*, 68).

20 Giordano, *Understanding Eating Disorders*, 71.

21 It should be noticed that if this is the case, the functional test should be able to detect any inability to use and weight information about food.

22 'Surgeon Defends Amputation', *BBC News*, 31 January 2000, http://news.bbc.co.uk/1/hi/scotland/625680.stm. For an argument against the demands of amputation by persons with BIID, see Daniel Patrone, 'Disfigured Anatomies and Imperfect Analogies: Body Integrity Identity Disorder and the Supposed Right to Self-Demanded Amputation of Healthy Body Parts', *Journal of Medical Ethics* 35, no. 9 (2009): 541–5. For a defence of the right to self-demanded amputation see Cristopher J. Ryan, 'Out on a Limb: The Ethical Management of Body Integrity Identity Disorder', *Neuroethics* 2, no. 1 (2009): 21–33.

23 Roberto Esposito, Filippo Cieri, Massimo di Giannantonio and Armando Tartaro, 'The Role of Body Image and Self-Perception in Anorexia Nervosa: The Neuroimaging Perspective', *Journal of Neuropsychology* 12, no. 1 (2016): 1–12.

24 Andrea Phillipou, Susan L. Rossell, Caroline Gurvich, David Jonathan Castle, Nikolaus F. Troje and Larry A. Abel, 'Body Image in Anorexia Nervosa: Body Size Estimation Utilising a Biological Motion Task and Eyetracking', *European Eating Disorders Review* 24, no. 2 (2016): 131–8.

25 Phillipou, Rossell, Gurvich, Castle, Troje and Abel, 'Body Image in Anorexia'; Esposito, Cieri, Giannantonio and Tartaro, 'The Role of Body Image and Self-Perception in Anorexia'; Panksepp and Biven, *Archeology of the Mind*; Giordano, *Understanding Eating Disorders*.

26 Giordano, *Understanding Eating Disorders*, 217, emphasis in original.

27 Bruch originally developed this argument. Recently, Duker and Slade have argued that the cognitive dysfunctions experienced by people with anorexia, especially those connected to food and eating, can be explained by brain damage and alterations caused by malnutrition. Bruch, *Eating Disorders*; Marilyn Duker and Roger Slade, *Anorexia and Bulimia: How to Help* (Buckingham: Open University Press, 2003).

28 See Chapter 6.

29 Karin Foerde, Joanna E. Steinglass, Daphna Shohamy and Timothy B. Walsh, 'Neural Mechanisms Supporting Maladaptive Food Choices in Anorexia Nervosa', *Nature Neuroscience* 18, no. 11 (2015): 1571–3.

30 Foerde, Steinglass, Shohamy and Walsh, 'Neural Mechanisms Supporting Maladaptive Food Choices'.

31 In Theroux's documentary on anorexia there is a young girl, Ifzana, who is having treatment against her will. She initially resists the therapy (e.g. she stands up for most of the time in order to burn calories), but thanks to the continuous care of medical staff she starts to be more engaged with the treatment and recognizes that her anorexic behaviour is not related to her authentic self. Ifzana affirms: 'I'm always in two minds I guess. The eating disorder part of me is obviously not thrilled, but the other side of me knows that it has to and I don't really have a choice.' Theroux, 'Talking to Anorexia'.

32 Wang, 'Mental Capacity Act'.

33 Giordano, *Understanding Eating Disorders*, 221, emphasis in original.

34 Here I stress the relevance accorded by English law to unwise and irrational desires. Within the MCA's functional and value-neutral approach, competent decisions are recognized by the correct *procedure* of thought applied and not by the *content* of the reasons and desires involved. From this point of view, there is no reason to discriminate anorexics' desire to maintain their 'unwise or irrational' relation with food. I will articulate this claim throughout the book.

35 Giordano calls her claim *brave* in opposition to Draper's account of anorexics' refusal of life-saving treatment. Draper affirms that anorexic's refusal can be considered competent if the refusal is grounded in judgements about her quality of life rather than on the basis of her fear of food or cognitive dysfunctions, but she does not specify if force-feeding is unjustifiable because it does not respect person's autonomy or because it can be a form of useless violence towards certain patients. According to Giordano, Draper avoids claiming that *all* competent patients' refusal should be respected due to her *precautionary* approach; according to Draper, the competent refusal of force-feeding should be respected only in *some* (unspecified) cases. Even while according to patients with anorexia the possibility of refusing treatment, Draper hares the prejudice of English law *presuming* that anorexia requires a different, *out of the norm* assessment; Giordano, *Understanding Eating Disorders*, 248–53; Heather Draper, 'Anorexia Nervosa and Respecting a Refusal of Life-Prolonging Therapy: A Limited Justification', *Bioethics* 14, no. 2 (2000): 120–33.

36 Giordano, *Understanding Eating Disorders*, 246, emphasis in original.

37 Giordano wrote her book *before* the application of the MCA (in the framework of the MHA); notwithstanding that, her critique of the legal approach towards anorexia remains valid.

38 Under the MCA the second option should be reformulated in this way: the second option is to show that patients experiencing anorexia lack capacity to decide about food due to their anorexia; Giordano, *Understanding Eating Disorders*, 197. Emphasis added.

39 Giordano, *Understanding Eating Disorders*, 193–4, emphasis added.

40 In a recent paper, in discussing a cross-national survey of physicians in Japan, the UK and the United States on how they assess decision-making capacity in patients with anorexia who refuse treatment, Takimoto arrives at the same conclusions advanced by Giordano. Yoshiyuki Takimoto, 'Key Components of the Mental Capacity Assessment of Patients with Anorexia Nervosa: A Study of Three Countries', *Journal of Eating Disorders* 10, no. 110 (2022): 1–10.

41 Takimoto, 'Key Components of the Mental Capacity', 54.

42 Takimoto, 'Key Components of the Mental Capacity', 48.

43 Diana T. Meyers, 'The Feminist Debate over Values in Autonomy Theory', in *Autonomy, Oppression, and Gender*, ed. Veltman and Piper, 116–20.

44 Meyers, 'Feminist Debate over Values', 116.

45 Meyers, 'Feminist Debate over Values', 120.

46 Andrea C. Westlund, 'Selflessness and Responsibility for Self: The Implications of Deference for Autonomy, Shared Agency and Love', *ProQuest Dissertations and Theses* (2001): 483–523; Andrea C. Westlund, 'Rethinking Relational Autonomy', *Hypatia* 24, no. 4 (2009): 26–49.

47 Meyers, 'Feminist Debate over Values', 126.

48 A reductive conception of capacities does not necessarily lead to a reduced conception of the *power* of certain particular capacities. The procedural approach reduces anorexics' power to decide on treatment, but it also strengthens and expands the power to formulate and defend procedural theories.

Chapter 3

1 Lord Donaldson, *Re T (Adult)* [1992] 4 All ER 649; see also *Sidaway (Appellant) v Bethlem Royal Hospital and the Maudsley Hospital Health Authority and Others* [1985] 1 All ER 643.

2 The functional test (MacCAT-T in English law) takes into account the sole procedural aspects of reasoning such as the capacity to understand and remember information, to use and weigh them and to communicate the decision. See Chapter 2.

3 Bernard Williams, *Moral Luck: Philosophical Papers 1973–1980* (Cambridge: Cambridge University Press, 1981).

4 Williams, *Moral Luck*, 101.

5 In a later paper, 'Internal Reasons and the Obscurity of Blame', Williams formulates the same point in a slightly different manner: B 'does not have a reason to drink what is in the [bottle], though he thinks he has. This is because there is not a *sound deliberative route* from his motivational set to this glass of petroleum: what he wants is a drink of gin and tonic.' Bernard Williams, *Making Sense of Humanity: And Other Philosophical Papers 1982–1993* (Cambridge: Cambridge University Press, 1995), 36.

6 David Hume, *A Treatise of Human Nature* (Oxford: Oxford University Press, 2000), 2.3.3.6.

7 Robert Brecher, *Getting What You Want? A Critique of Liberal Morality* (London: Routledge, 1997), 42.

8 Rationality, on this view, 'is the following of perceived self-interest'. Philippa Foot, 'Does Moral Subjectivism Rest on a Mistake?', *Oxford Journal of Legal Studies* 15, no. 1 (1995): 1–14, 6.

9 Alan H. Goldman, 'Reason Internalism', *Philosophy and Phenomenological Research* 71, no. 3 (2005): 505–32.

10 The alternative, for Williams, and more generally for the internalist, is to ground the moral demands in some sort of human empathy.

11 I use the term 'liberalism' in a very broad sense, referring to all those political and philosophical approaches that understand the idea of *right* (domain of *justice*) as prior to and independent of the idea of the *good* (the domain of *morality* and *ethics*).

12 'Fabian Freyenhagen – the Philosophical Terrain', YouTube video, posted by EssexAutonomyProject, 26 April 2012, https://www.youtube.com/watch?v=F4-B6JH91dM.

13 'An adult patient who … suffers from no mental incapacity has an absolute right to choose whether to consent to medical treatment … This right of choice is not limited to decisions which others might regard as sensible. It exists notwithstanding that the reasons for making the choice are rational, irrational, unknown or even nonexistent.' *Re T (Adult: Refusal of Medical Treatment),* (1992).

14 The capacity to 'use' and 'weigh' information during the process of decision-making is understood in terms of cognitive processes. Given the reasons and the values that the person accepts, the capacity to use information is positively assessed if the reasoning applied can be interpreted as a correct series of inferences. Making a decision is not properly a question of 'reasoning' but more a question of making a procedurally correct 'use' of the information. As Owen underlines, the semantic choice of the verbs 'use' and 'weigh' and the omission of the term 'reason' in the MCA is indicative of the radical disassociation in UK law between rationality and mental capacity. An alternative formulation – developed by Grisso and Applebaum, and adopted in the United States – states instead that what has to be assessed is 'the ability to *reason* with the relevant information so as to engage in a logical process of weighing treatment options'. According to the MCA, mental capacity is structurally dissociated from rationality, and the only reasons and norms that can be presupposed in the assessment of decisional capacity are those accepted by the person: Gareth S. Owen, Fabian Freyenhagen, Genevra Richardson and Matthew Hotopf, 'Mental Capacity and Decisional Autonomy: An Interdisciplinary Challenge', *Inquiry* 52, no. 1 (2009): 79–107; T. Grisso and P. S. Appelbaum, *Assessing Competence to Consent to Treatment: A Guide for Physicians and Other Health Professionals* (Oxford: Oxford University Press, 1998). Emphasis added.

15 See Chapter 2

16 Williams, *Moral Luck*, 101.

17 Williams, *Moral Luck*, 106, emphasis in original.

18 Williams, *Moral Luck*, 107.

19 Williams, *Moral Luck*, 107.

20 David Sobel, 'Explanation, Internalism, and Reasons for Action', *Social Philosophy and Policy* 18, no. 2 (2001): 218–35.

21 For a broader perspective on externalism see Adam Carter, Jesper Kallestrup, Orestis S. Palermos and Duncan Pritchard, 'Varieties of Externalism', *Philosophical Issues* 24, no. 1 (2014): 63–109.

22 For a more fine-grained internalist critique of externalism see Goldman, 'Reason Internalism'.

23 For a defence of this approach, see Sarah Conly, *Against Autonomy: Justifying Coercive Paternalism* (Cambridge: Cambridge University Press, 2013).

24 'Every man has a "property" in his own "person". This nobody has a right to, but himself.' John Locke, *The Second Treatise on Civil Government* (New Haven: Yale University Press, 2003), chap. V, §26.

25 According to Richard Norman, the appeal to the concept of motivation derives from the assumption of a misleading picture of the agent: 'The picture is of human beings as essentially static, beings whose natural condition is one of inaction, and who need some kind of motivating force to effect the transition from inaction to action.' Norman instead suggests that 'as long as we are conscious, and not asleep, under a general anaesthetic, comatose or dead … we are always acting'. From this point of view, the concept of motivation becomes redundant because it does not add anything to reasons; there are no reasons for acting, but only reasons for doing something instead of something else.

> Insofar as we are rational beings we just *do* act on our beliefs about what we have reasons to do. If A believes that he has a good reason to φ, and he does φ, nothing else is needed to bridge the gap between his believing he has the reason and his φ-ing, or between his believing he has the reasons and his being motivated to φ (Richard Norman, 'Practical Reasons and the Redundancy of Motives', *Ethical Theory and Moral Practice* 4 (2001): 3–22)

26 Tan, Hope and Stewart, 'Anorexia Nervosa and Personal Identity'; Hope, Tan, Stewart and Fitzpatrick, 'Anorexia and the Language of Authenticity'; Hope, Tan, Stewart and McMillan, 'Agency, Ambivalence and Authenticity'.

27 See Chapter 1.

28 Saukko, *The Anorexic Self*; Giordano, *Understanding Eating Disorders*; Tan, 'Competence to Make Treatment Decisions in Anorexia'; Hope, Tan, Stewart and Fitzpatrick, 'Anorexia and the Language of Authenticity'.

29 Hope, Tan, Stewart and Fitzpatrick, 'Anorexia and the Language of Authenticity'.

30 See Chapter 1.

31 Paul Benson, 'Free Agent and Self-Worth', *Journal of Philosophy* 91, no. 12 (1994): 656–7.

32 Benson draws his example from George Cukor's movie *Gaslight* (1944):

> Ingrid Bergman plays a character married to an evil man, played by Charles Boyer. The Boyer character has murdered Bergman's aunt and has married Bergman just so that he can find and steal the valuable jewels that the aunt hid before her death. Bergman, who knows none of this, believes that her husband really loves her. Boyer's scheme is to reduce Bergman to a state of such apparent confusion and disorientation that she will be unlikely to realize what he is up to. He isolates her from other people, not by force but through suggestions that seem innocent enough to Bergman. He makes her think that she is losing things, that she cannot remember things she recently has done, that she is subject to hallucinations. (Benson, 'Free Agent and Self-Worth', 655)

33 Andrew D. Spear, 'Epistemic Dimension of Gaslighting: Peer-Disagreement, Self-Trust, and Epistemic Injustice', *Inquiry* 66, no. 1 (2019): 68–91.

34 I analyse the relation between oppressive social contexts and autonomy in Chapter 4.

35 Levin offers this line of reasoning: 'Whether the assignment of sex roles is a device to keep women in thrall depends on how this assignment came about and how it is sustained. It is not an oppressive device if it came about because men and women for the most part innately prefer things the way they are, or as an unintended consequence of preferences.' Michael Levin, *Feminism and Freedom* (New Brunswick: Transaction Books, 1987), 38.

36 The philosophical roots of this idea can be found in Hume:

> Since reason alone can never produce any action, or give rise to volition, I infer that the same faculty is as incapable of preventing volition, or of disputing the preference with any passion or emotion … Nothing can oppose or retard the impulse of passion, but a contrary impulse; and if this contrary impulse ever arises from reason, that latter faculty must have an original influence on the will, and must be able to cause, as well as hinder any act of volition … Reason is, and ought only to be the slave of the passions, and can never pretend to any other office than to serve and obey them … A passion is an original existence, or, if you will, modification of existence, and contains not any representative quality, which renders it a copy of any other existence or modification. When I am angry, I am actually possest with the passion, and in that emotion have no more a reference to any other object, than when I am thirsty, or sick, or more than five foot high. 'Tis impossible, therefore, that this passion can be oppos'd by, or be contradictory to truth and reason; since this contradiction consists in the disagreement of ideas, consider'd as copies, with those objects, which they represent. (Hume, *Treatise on Human Nature*, 2.3.3.5)

37 George H. Mead, *Mind, Self and Society* (Chicago: University of Chicago Press, 1934).

38 Charles Taylor, 'Politics of Recognition', in *Multiculturalism: Examining the Politics of Recognition*, ed. Emy Gutmann (Princeton: Princeton University Press, 1994), 32–3, emphasis in original.

39 Susan Wolf, *Freedom within Reason* (New York: Oxford University Press, 1990), 75.

40 Hope, Tan, Stewart and Fitzpatrick, 'Anorexia and the Language of Authenticity'.

41 There is no single 'liberal' point of view, and within the liberal tradition it is possible to find different interpretations of the relation between autonomy and paternalism. For a clarification on my use of the term 'liberalism', see note 11.

42 Kant's 'Dare to know!' is aimed at atomic individuals, we might say.

43 Macpherson claims that the private conception of motivations and desires is the source of the political and ethical problems of liberalism: 'The difficulties of modern liberal-democratic theory lies … in its conception of the individual as essentially the proprietor of his own person or capacities, owing nothing to society for them. The individual [is] seen neither as a moral whole, nor as a part of a larger social whole, but as an owner of himself.' For an in-depth analysis of the private conception of reasons endorsed by liberalism, see Brecher (1997): 'For something to count as a reason for an action, it has to have some conceivable justificatory connection with that action. I can no more think that just anything can constitute a reason "for me" than I can want just anything at all: there has to be a context within which its constituting a reason in conceivable.' Crawford B. Macpherson, *The Political Theory of Possessive Individualism* (Oxford: Oxford University Press, 1962), 3; Brecher, *Getting What You Want?*, 104.

44 Charles Taylor, *Philosophical Papers 1: Human Agency and Language* (Cambridge: Cambridge University Press, 1985), 215–92; Charles Taylor, *Philosophical Arguments* (Cambridge: Harvard University Press, 1995), 61–78, 79–99, 165–80.

45 More precisely, in *Sources of the Self*, as well as in *The Ethics of Authenticity*, Taylor investigates the sources of the concept of the self, especially regarding its relation with the ideal – born at the end of the eighteenth century, and based on the conceptions of individualism that arose in the seventeenth century – of authenticity. On Taylor's view, the concept of autonomy, as well as the concept of freedom, is articulated on the ground of the relation between the self and the ideal of authenticity; in very general terms, being autonomous means essentially being able (and being allowed) to be oneself. For the sake of my argument, I shall make reference to a monological conception of autonomy even if Taylor does not use this precise formulation. Charles Taylor, *Philosophy and the Human Sciences. Philosophical Papers 2* (Cambridge: Cambridge University Press, 1985); Charles Taylor, *Sources of Self. The Making of the Modern Identity* (Harvard: Harvard University Press, 1989); Charles Taylor, *The Ethics of Authenticity* (Harvard: Harvard University Press, 2003).

46 Taylor, *Philosophical Arguments*, 7.

47 I shall deepen this point in the Chapter 4.

48 Taylor, *The Ethics of Authenticity*, 47–8, emphasis in original.

49 From a wittgensteinian perspective, the questions '*What* do we want when we aim at something nonsensical?' and '*Why* we aim at something nonsensical?' are basically the same. The understanding of a contradictory approach to reality corresponds to the disappearance of the (alleged) motive underlying it; or, in other words, the acknowledgment of a contradiction is inseparable from the liberation from its influence (and from the idea that there is a *content* in the nonsense). James Conant, 'Elucidation and Nonsense in Frege and Early Wittgenstein', in *The New Wittgenstein*, ed. Alice Crary and Rupert Read (London: Routledge, 2000), 174–218.

50 Paul Benson, 'Feminist Commitments and Relational Autonomy', in Veltman and Piper, *Autonomy, Oppression, and Gender*, 109.

51 Westlund, 'Rethinking Relational Autonomy'.

52 Benson, 'Feminist Commitments and Relational Autonomy'.

Chapter 4

1 Lorrain Code, *What Can She Know? Feminist Theory and the Construction of Knowledge* (Ithaca: Cornell University Press, 1991), 78.

2 Alison M. Jaggar, *Feminist Politics and Human Nature* (Totowa: Rowman & Allanheld, 1983), 47–8.

3 Jaggar, *Feminist Politics and Human Nature*, 47–8.

4 Code, *What Can She Know?*, 78.

5 Mackenzie and Stoljar, *Relational Autonomy*, 3–4.

6 Charles Taylor, *The Language Animal: The Full Shape of the Human Linguistic Capacity* (Cambridge, MA: Harvard University Press, 2016); Taylor, *Sources of Self*; Amartya K. Sen, *The Idea of Justice* (London: Penguin, 2010); Alasdair MacIntyre, *After Virtue* (Notre Dame: University of Notre Dame Press, 1988).

7 As I will show in this chapter, some scholars think that interpersonal relations and social contexts are necessary only for the development of autonomy, while others claim that this applies also to its maintenance and exercise.

8 Cora Diamond, 'Losing Your Concepts', *Ethics* 98, no. 2 (1988): 255–77; Taylor, *Sources of Self*; Taylor, *Ethics of Authenticity*.

9 Taylor, *Philosophical Arguments*, 127–45; Amartya K. Sen, *Development as Freedom* (Oxford: Oxford University Press, 1999); Martha Nussbaum, 'Symposium on Amartya Sen's Philosophy: 5 Adaptive Preferences and Women's Options', *Economics and Philosophy* 17, no. 1 (2001): 67–88.

10 This conception is generally labelled *negative* conception of freedom; it contrasts with a *positive* conception of liberty. Isaiah Berlin, 'Two Concepts of Liberty', in *Liberty: Incorporating Four Essays on Liberty*, ed. Isaiah Berlin (Oxford: Oxford University Press, 2002), 166–217.

11 Mackenzie and Stoljar, *Relational Autonomy*, 21–2; Veltman and Piper, *Autonomy, Oppression, and Gender*, 2–3.

12 Ann E. Cudd, 'Oppression by Choice', *Journal of Social Philosophy* 25, no. 1 (1994): 22–44.

13 Mackenzie and Stoljar, *Relational Autonomy*, 3–5.

14 Westlund, 'Rethinking Relational Autonomy', 35.

15 Paul Benson, 'Taking Ownership: Authority and Voice in Autonomous Agency', in *Autonomy and the Challenges of Liberalism: New Essays*, ed. Joel Anderson and John Christman (Cambridge: Cambridge University Press, 2005), 101–26; Benson, 'Free Agency'; Carolyn McLeod, 'Relational Autonomy, Self-Trust and Health Care for Patients Who Are Oppressed', in Mackenzie and Stoljar, *Relational Autonomy*.

16 Veltman and Piper, *Autonomy, Oppression, and Gender*, 3.

17 Veltman and Piper, *Autonomy, Oppression, and Gender*, 3.

18 Jon Elster, *Sour Grapes: Studies in the Subversion of Rationality* (Cambridge: Cambridge University Press, 1983); S. J. Khader, *Adaptive Preferences and Women's Empowerment* (Oxford: Oxford University Press, 2011).

19 Cudd, 'Oppression by Choice'; Ann E. Cudd, *Analyzing Oppression* (Oxford: Oxford University Press, 2006).

20 The title of the book *Sour Grapes* – Jon Elster's pioneering study on adaptive preference formation – is a reference to the Aesop's fable *The Fox and the Grapes*. In this fable, a fox wants to eat some grapes on a vine, but he cannot reach them. Instead of acknowledging that he cannot attain them, he claims that they are unwanted because due to their sourness.

21 Marina Oshana, 'A Commitment to Autonomy Is a Commitment to Feminism', in Veltman and Piper, *Autonomy, Oppression, and Gender*, 152; Marina Oshana, *Personal Autonomy and Social Oppression* (New York: Routledge, 2015); Natalie Stoljar, 'Autonomy and the Feminist Intuition', in Mackenzie and Stoljar, *Relational Autonomy*, 95; Natalie Stoljar, 'Autonomy and Adaptive Preference Formation', in Veltman and Piper, *Autonomy, Oppression, and Gender*.

22 Alfred Mele, *Autonomous Agents: From Self-Control to Autonomy* (Oxford: Oxford University Press, 1995); Marilyn Friedman, *Autonomy, Gender, Politics* (Oxford: Oxford University Press, 2003), 5, 96, 146, 152–9; John Christman, *The Politics of Persons: Individual Autonomy and Socio-Historical Selves* (Cambridge: Cambridge University Press, 2009), 155–6.

23 Mackenzie and Stoljar, *Relational Autonomy*, 4, emphasis added.

24 Oshana, 'Commitment to Autonomy'.

25 Mackenzie and Stoljar, *Relational Autonomy*.

26 Kristin Luker, *Taking Choices: Abortion and the Decision Not to Contracept* (Berkeley: University of California Press, 1975).

27 Mackenzie and Stoljar, *Relational Autonomy*, 98, 109.

28 Diana Meyers, 'Feminism and Women's Autonomy: The Challenge of Female Genital Cutting', *Metaphilosophy* 31, no. 5 (2000): 469–91.

29 Meyers, 'Feminism and Women's Autonomy'.

30 John Christman, 'Relational Autonomy, Liberal Individualism, and the Social Construction of Selves', *Philosophical Studies* 117, nos. 1–2 (2004): 143–64.

31 Paul Benson, 'Feminist Intuitions and the Normative Substance of Autonomy', in *Personal Autonomy: New Essays on Personal Autonomy and Its Role in Contemporary Moral Philosophy*, ed. James S. Taylor (Cambridge: Cambridge University Press, 2005), 124–42.

32 Christman, 'Relational Autonomy, Liberal Individualism', 153.

33 John Christman, 'Coping or Oppression: Autonomy and Adaptation to Circumstance', in Veltman and Piper, *Autonomy, Oppression, and Gender*, 221.

34 Christman takes into account both the effective reflections operated by the agent during the period of the development of the motivational set and the retrospective reflections that the agent can make if she was too young (or unaware) during that period; Christman, *The Politics of Persons*, 155–6.

35 John Christman, 'Autonomy and Personal History', *Canadian Journal of Philosophy* 21, no. 1 (1991): 1–24.

36 On the same lines, Marilyn Friedman writes that a woman who 'chooses or acts in accord with wants or desired that she has self-reflectively endorsed … is behaving autonomously'; Friedman, *Autonomy, Gender, Politics*, 5.

37 Christman, 'Relational Autonomy, Liberal Individualism', 154.

38 Friedman, *Autonomy, Gender, Politics*, 152–9.

39 Friedman, *Autonomy, Gender, Politics*, 152.

40 Benson, 'Autonomy and Oppressive Socialization'; Marina Oshana, *Personal Autonomy and Society* (London: Routledge, 2006).

41 Catriona Mackenzie, 'Three Dimensions of Autonomy: A Relational Analysis', in Veltman and Piper, *Autonomy, Oppression, and Gender*, 20.

42 Catriona Mackenzie, Wendy Rogers and Susan Dodds, 'Introduction: What Is Vulnerability, and Why Does It Matter for Moral Theory?', in *Vulnerability: New Essays in Ethics and Feminist Philosophy*, ed. Catriona Mackenzie, Wendy Rogers and Susan Dodds (Oxford: Oxford University Press, 2014), 1.

43 Mackenzie proposes a taxonomy of three, and not two, sources of vulnerability, but for now I will take into account only the first two since the third – *pathogenic* sources of vulnerability, regarding the vulnerability caused by interpersonal relationships and institutions – can be considered as a specification of the second – *situational*, context-dependent sources of vulnerability. Furthermore, it is important to underline that this differentiation of sources of vulnerability is not a categorical distinction but a way of identifying 'the variety and context – specificity of sources of vulnerability, … [the] responsibilities owed to the 'more than ordinarily vulnerable, and the potential interventions to mitigate the effects of various forms of vulnerability'. Mackenzie, Rogers and Dodds, *Vulnerability*, 7–8.

44 Mackenzie, Rogers and Dodds, *Vulnerability*.

45 Alasdair MacIntyre, *Dependent Rational Animals: Why Human Beings Need the Virtues* (Chicago: Open Court, 1999), 8, 49, 81.

46 MacIntyre, *Dependent Rational Animals*, 8.

47 For an analysis of the manner in which the conditions imposed by vulnerability are avoided by liberal philosophers, see Martha Nussbaum, *Hiding from Humanity: Disgust, Shame, and the Law* (Princeton: Princeton University Press, 2004); for an analysis of the empiricist approach to disembodied rationality, see Taylor, *The Language Animal*.

48 MacIntyre, *Dependent Rational Animals*, 8.

49 MacIntyre, *Dependent Rational Animals*, 81.

50 Mackenzie, Rogers and Dodds, *Vulnerability*, 7.

51 Mackenzie, Rogers and Dodds, *Vulnerability*, 38.

52 Mackenzie, Rogers and Dodds, *Vulnerability*, 39.

53 Mackenzie, Rogers and Dodds, *Vulnerability*, 16–17, emphasis added.

54 Catriona Mackenzie, 'The Importance of Relational Autonomy and Capabilities for an Ethics of Vulnerability', in *Vulnerability: New Essays in Ethics and Feminist Philosophy*, ed. Catriona Mackenzie, Wendy Rogers and Susan Dodds (Oxford: Oxford University Press, 2014).

55 Mackenzie, Rogers and Dodds, *Vulnerability*, 35.

56 Mackenzie and Stoljar, *Relational Autonomy*, 22.

57 Friedman, *Autonomy, Gender, Politics*, 96.

58 Mackenzie and Stoljar, *Relational Autonomy*, 23.

59 Katrina Hutchison, Catriona Mackenzie and Marina Oshana, *Social Dimensions of Moral Responsibility* (Oxford: Oxford University Press, 2018), 12.

60 The relation between oppression and autonomy is differently interpreted by defenders of constitutive approaches to autonomy, and its assessment usually depends on the typology of values assumed by the theory. Constitutive conceptions incorporating strong substantivism are keener to directly deduce heteronomy from oppression, while notions subsuming weak substantivism are more concerned with investigating the state of agents' self-regarding attitudes and dialogical capacities within contexts of oppression. For a constitutively relational conception based on strong substantivism, see Oshana, *Personal Autonomy and Society*. For a constitutively relational notion grounded in weak substantivism, see Benson, 'Free Agent and Self-Worth'.

61 Lorrain Code, 'The Perversion of Autonomy and the Subjection of Women: Discourses of Social Advocacy at Century's End', in *Relational Autonomy: Feminist Perspectives on Autonomy, Agency, and the Social Self*, ed. Catriona Mackenzie and Natalie Stoljar (Oxford: Oxford University Press, 2000), 185–6.

62 Marina Oshana, 'Personal Autonomy and Society', *Canadian Journal of Philosophy* 29, no. 1 (1998), 81–102.

63 John Christman admits that normatively neutral accounts of autonomy cannot be disconnected by values, but he explains this relation from a causal, and not constitutive, point of view: 'Certain value commitments are required for autonomy because the core conditions of autonomy (reflective, competent, self-acceptance) cannot be *achieved* without those commitments *but not because such commitments are inherently valid or justified*.' Emphasis added; Christman, 'Coping or Oppression', 216.

64 Benson, 'Free Agent and Self-Worth'.

65 Taylor, *Philosophical Papers 1*, 209.

66 Taylor, *Philosophical Arguments*, 92–9.

67 Taylor, *Philosophical Arguments*, 181–203.

68 Friedman, *Autonomy, Gender, Politics*, 146.

69 Christman, 'Coping or Oppression', 221.

70 Christman, 'Autonomy and Personal History'.

71 Christman, 'Coping or Oppression', 217–18, emphasis added.

72 Paul Benson, 'Autonomy and Oppressive Socialization', *Social Theory and Practice* 17, no. 3 (1991): 403.

73 The literature on autonomy and adaptive preferences tackles similar problems to the literature on ideology and false consciousness. Both are focused on the relation between agency and oppression, but while the latter is interested in the role of material, ideological, cultural and institutional factors in the agent's self-understanding, the former is concerned with the function of options available for the development of preferences. I have decided to dedicate more space to the literature on adaptive preferences because, on the one hand, I aim to criticize the MCA on the basis of its understanding of autonomy – which is articulated in terms of choices and preferences, more than of identity and reasons – and, on the other hand, because I aim to analyse and highlight the function of ideology by investigating the wider role of language and dialogicity for autonomy. Uma Narayan, 'Minds of Their Own: Choices, Practices, Autonomy, and Other Women', in *A Mind of One's Own: Feminist Essays on Reason and Objectivity*, ed. Louise M. Antony and Charlotte E. Witt (London: Routledge, 2002), 418–32.

74 Mackenzie, Rogers and Dodds, *Vulnerability*, 37–9.

75 Diamond, 'Losing Your Concepts'; Stanley Cavell, *Condition Handsome and Unhandsome: The Constitution of Emersonian Perfectionism. The Carus Lectures 1988* (Chicago: University of Chicago Press, 1990), 101–26; Charles Taylor, *Dilemmas and Connections* (Cambridge, MA: Harvard University Press, 2011), 39–55.

76 Christman, 'Coping or Oppression', 209.

77 Elster, *Sour Grapes*; Benson, 'Autonomy and Oppressive Socialization'; Benson, 'Feminist Commitments and Relational Autonomy'; Nussbaum, 'Symposium on Amartya Sen's Philosophy'; Oshana, *Personal Autonomy and Society*; M. Vargas, 'The Social Constitution of Agency and Responsibility: Oppression, Politics, and Moral Ecology', in *Social Dimensions of Moral Responsibility*, ed. Katrina Hutchison, Catriona Mackenzie and Marina Oshana (Oxford: Oxford University Press, 2018), 110–36.

78 In a recent article, Laura Sullivan and Fay Niker argue that relational conceptions of autonomy have opened a new conceptual space for a reconfiguration of the concept of paternalism. In their view, relational notions of autonomy allow an understanding of interpersonal intervention that does not presuppose the idea of interference because, within the relational framework, 'our choices are already influenced by and dependent on the acts of others'. In their view, 'interventions [based on relational conceptions of autonomy] fall outside the bounds of paternalism, meaning that attempts to describe them using the conceptual framework of paternalism will misconstrue their ethically salient features and may misjudge their ethical justification. To describe these interventions, we propose using the conceptual framework of maternalism.' Laura S. Sullivan and Fay Niker, 'Relational Autonomy, Paternalism, and Maternalism', *Ethical Theory and Moral Practice* 21, no. 3 (2018): 655.

79 Mackenzie, Rogers and Dodds, *Vulnerability*, 35.

Chapter 5

1 Robert B. Brandom, *Making It Explicit* (Cambridge, MA: Harvard University Press, 1998); Benson, 'Taking Ownership'; Westlund, 'Rethinking Relational Autonomy'.

2 Benson, 'Feminist Commitments'.

3 Meyers, 'The Feminist Debate over Values'.

4 Taylor, *Philosophical Papers 1*, 97–114; Taylor, *Philosophical Arguments*, 61–78; Charles Taylor, *A Secular Age* (Cambridge, MA: Harvard University Press, 2007), 539–93.

5 Taylor and Dreyfus, *Retrieving Realism*, 20.

6 Meyers, 'The Feminist Debate over Values'.

7 Many thinkers trace back the value-saturated notion of autonomy to Kant, but I think this is rather reductive. See Immanuel Kant, 'Dignity and Self-Respect', in *Lectures on Ethics*, ed. Immanuel Kant, trans. Louis Infield (New York: Harper & Row, 1963); Immanuel Kant, *Grounding for the Metaphysics of Morals*, trans. Mary Gregor (Indianapolis: Hackett Publishing Company, 1981). For a value-saturated notion of autonomy grounded in Kant, see Anita Superson, 'Deformed Desires and Informed Desire Tests', *Hypatia* 20, no. 4 (2005): 109–26. For a defence of a more nuanced notion of Kantian autonomy, see Brecher, *Getting What You Want?*; Robert Brecher, 'Why the Kantian Ideal Survives Medical Learning Curves, and Why It Matters', *Journal of Medical Ethics* 32, no. 9 (2006): 511–12.

8 Susan J. Brison, 'Relational Autonomy and Freedom of Expression', in Mackenzie and Stoljar, *Relational Autonomy*, 280–300.

9 See Chapters 3 and 4.

10 Taylor, *Philosophical Arguments*, 76.

11 Taylor, *The Language Animal*, 108.

12 John Locke, *An Essay Concerning Human Understanding* (London: Penguin Books, 1998), book 3.

13 Taylor, *Philosophical Arguments*, 74.

14 Étienne B. de Condillac, *Essay on the Origin of Human Knowledge* (Cambridge: Cambridge University Press, 2001), 113–22.

15

> When they (my elders) named some object, and accordingly moved towards something, I saw this and I grasped that the thing was called by the sound they uttered when they meant to point it out. Their intention was shown by their bodily movements, as it were the natural language of all peoples: the expression of the face, the play of the eyes, the movement of other parts of the body, and the tone of voice which expresses our state of mind in seeking, having, rejecting, or avoiding something. Thus, as I heard words repeatedly used in their proper places in various sentences, I gradually learnt to understand what objects they signified; and after I had trained my mouth to form these signs, I used them to express my own desires. (Augustine, *Confessions*, trans. Henry Chadwick (Oxford: Oxford University Press, 1998), I.8)

16 Ludwig Wittgenstein, *Philosophical Investigations*, trans. Gertrude E. M. Anscombe (London: Wiley-Blackwell, 2009), §32.

17 Taylor, *Philosophical Papers 1*, 228–9.

18 Taylor, *Philosophical Arguments*, 79–99.

19 Johann G. von Herder, *On the Origin of Language*, trans. John H. Moran and Alexander Gode (Chicago: University of Chicago Press, 1986).

20 Taylor, *Philosophical Papers 1*, 83–4.

21 Taylor, *Philosophical Papers 1*, 23; Taylor, *Philosophical Papers 2*, 3–4; Taylor, *Philosophical Arguments*, 96–7; Taylor, *The Ethics of Authenticity*, 260–1.

22 Wittgenstein, *Philosophical Investigations*, §30.

23 Tomasello argues that the crucial difference between the ostensive gesture of the big apes and humans relies on the fact that humans interact in the domain of a relational activity characterized by a set of common purposes and joint attention: 'Human cooperative communication is more complex than ape intentional communication because its underlying social-cognitive infrastructure comprises not only skills for understanding individual intentionality but also skills and motivations for shared intentionality.' Advanced primates can identify the intentions of their conspecifics, but only humans can understand and imitate others' *communicative* intentions. Tomasello, *Origins of Human Communication*, 321. See also Melvin Konner, *The Evolution of Childhood* (Cambridge, MA: Harvard University Press, 2010), chapter 19.

24 Wittgenstein, *Philosophical Investigations*, §199.

25 I am not aiming to offer a thorough 'list' of the conditions required for the understanding of ostensive definitions (as I shall explain further, such an enterprise would be inconclusive by definition). My only aim here is to claim that such an understanding *is grounded* in these kind of conditions.

26 The idea that singular words have meaning only within the domain of a contrastive language is defined by Taylor as *holism of meaning*. One of the most influential forms of this idea can be found in De Saussure: 'In language there are differences *without positive terms*. Whether we take the signified or the signifier, language has neither ideas nor sounds that existed before the linguistic system.' Ferdinand de Saussure, *Course in General Linguistics* (New York: Philosophical Library, 1959), 120, emphasis in original; Wittgenstein, *Philosophical Investigations*, §30.

27 There is no doubt that Wittgenstein is not only aware that the question is badly formulated, but also that he is asking the wrong question for a reason. He thinks that we can remain entangled in some misguiding or ineffective ways of using language, and that when this happens, we become unable to understand what makes our questions and assertions senseless. In a way, certain forms of expressions, certain ways of talking about the world and ourselves, become part of who we are, and it becomes very difficult not only to overcome the impediment and achieve more effective uses of language but also to simply recognize that 'a *picture* held us captive'. Wittgenstein's use of senseless questions and assertions is directed precisely to the peculiar kind of difficulties we meet when we try to understand (or help) someone who utters nonsense.

28 According to Wittgenstein, a senseless question or statement can always become sensible if it is contextualized and if its constituent terms are made intelligible. In this case, we could do that by looking at the 'what' of the question as referring to a background of partially articulated assumptions instead of a strictly articulated definition.

29 Taylor, *Philosophical Arguments*, 68–9.

30 Even if, in practice, humans are generally able to operate with the background required for language, communication is inevitably fallible and its efficacy cannot be simply presupposed. For an interesting analysis of this topic and its relation with scepticism, see Cavell, *Condition Handsome and Unhandsome*.

31 'Ask yourself whether our own language is complete – whether it was so before the symbolism of chemistry and the notation of the infinitesimal calculus were incorporated in to it: for these are, so to speak, suburbs of our language. (And how many houses or streets does it take before a town begins to be a town?).' Wittgenstein, *Philosophical Investigations*, §18.

32 Wittgenstein, *Philosophical Investigations*, 69.

33 'Giving grounds, however, justifying the evidence, comes to an end; but the end is not certain propositions' striking us immediately as true, i.e. it is not a kind of *seeing* on our part; it is our *acting*, which lies at the bottom of the language-game.' Wittgenstein, *Philosophical Investigations*, § 204, emphasis in original.

34 In this case, my articulation of the background is motivated by elucidatory purposes. The term 'elucidation' is notoriously used by Wittgenstein in one of the very last sentences of the *Tractatus*: 'My propositions serve as *elucidations* in the following

way: anyone who understands me eventually recognizes them as *nonsensical,* when he has used them – as steps – to climb out through them, on them, over them. (He must, so to speak, throw away the ladder after he has climbed up it.)' It is important to underline that even if the *Tractatus*' sentences cannot be understood without being 'thrown away', this does apply to every articulation of the background:

> The proposition describing the [background] might be part of a kind of mythology. And their role is like that of rules of game; and the game can be learned purely practically, without leaning any explicit rule. It might be imagined that some propositions, of the form of empirical propositions, were hardened and functioned as channels for such empirical propositions as were not hardened but fluid; and that this relation altered with time, in that fluid propositions hardened, and hard ones became fluid. The mythology may change back into a state of flux, the river-bed of thoughts may shift. But I distinguish between the movement of the waters on the river-bed and the shift of the bed itself; though there is not a sharp division of the one from the other. (Ludwig Wittgenstein, *Tractatus Logico-Philosophicus*, trans. D. F. Pears and B. F. McGuinness (London: Routledge, 2001), §6.54; Ludwig Wittgenstein, *On Certainty*, trans. Denis Paul and Gertrude E. M. Anscombe (Oxford: Basil Blackwell, 1969), §95–7).

35 Taylor, *Philosophical Arguments*, 96.

36 This conception of language belongs to a long and influential philosophical tradition that can be seen as grounded – at least in its 'modern' version – in the representational or monological epistemology constructed by Descartes. As Taylor puts it,

> Words are given meaning by being attached to the things represented via the 'ideas' which represent them. The introduction of words greatly facilitates the combinations of ideas into responsible picture. This facilitation is understood in different ways. For Hobbes and Locke, they allow us to grasp things in classes, and hence make possible synthesis wholesale where nonlinguistic intuition would be confined to the painstaking association of particulars. Condillac thinks that the introduction of language gives us for the first time control over the whole process of association; it affords us 'dominion over our imagination'. (Taylor, *The Language Animal*, 4–5)

Modern and contemporary empiricists generally defend this conception of language, but it is also shared – among others – by behaviourists like Skinner, and by defenders of an account of meaning in terms of truth-conditions such as Davidson, Rorty and Quine. See René Descartes, *Discourse on Method and Meditations on First* Philosophy, trans. Donald A. Cress (Indianapolis: Hackett, 1998), 11; Thomas Hobbes, *Leviathan* (Oxford: Blackwell, 1989), 20; Locke, *Essay Concerning Human Understanding*; Condillac, *Essay on the Origin of Human Knowledge*; Donald Davidson, 'Radical Interpretation', *Dialectica* 27, nos. 3–4 (1973): 313–28; Willard V. Quine, 'Epistemology Naturalized', in *Ontological Relativity and Other Essays* (New York: Columbia University Press, 1969); Richard Rorty, *Philosophy and the Mirror of Nature* (Princeton: Princeton University Press, 1979); Quentin Skinner, 'Language and Political Change', in *Political Innovation and Conceptual Change*, ed. Quentin Skinner

(Cambridge: Cambridge University Press, 1989), 6–23; Taylor, *Ethics of Authenticity*, 143–77; Taylor, *Philosophical Papers 1*, 248–92.

37 Taylor, *Philosophical Arguments*, 96. Emphasis added. See also Wittgenstein, *Philosophical Investigations*, §23.

38 Wittgenstein, *Philosophical Investigations*, 97.

39 Wittgenstein, *Philosophical Investigations*, 256–9, emphasis added.

40 'But I did not get my picture of the world by satisfying myself of its correctness; nor do I have it because I am satisfied of its correctness. No: it is the *inherited* background against which I distinguish between true and false.' Wittgenstein, *On Certainty*, §94, emphasis added.

41 Wittgenstein, *Philosophical Investigations*, §241.

42 Wittgenstein's later texts are characterized by the presence of multiple, contrasting 'voices'. For this reason, many scholars – Wittgenstein included – have compared his texts to Plato's dialogues. On the one hand, Wittgenstein's later texts contain a lot of assertions and questions that are in disagreement with his view or that are grounded in a misunderstanding of his arguments (as the affirmation quoted here). Like Plato's dialogues, the presence of these 'antagonistic' views allows a dialogical process that leads to an articulation of the arguments that directly face the assumptions at the basis of the different points of view animating the dialogue. On the other hand, however, Wittgenstein's standpoint is 'antithetical to the one occupied by Socrates in the Platonic dialogues'. In the words of Wittgenstein, 'If I were asked what knowledge is, I would enumerate instances of knowledge and add the words "and similar things". There is no shared constituent to be discovered in them since none exists.' Ludwig Wittgenstein, 'Dictation for Schlick', in *The Voices of Wittgenstein: The Vienna Circle. Ludwig Wittgenstein and Friedrich Waismann*, ed. Gordon Baker (London: Routledge, 2003): 30. According to Wittgenstein, the 'similarities overlapping and criss-crossing' different uses of the same word (e.g. 'knowledge') do not depend on a common essence underlying the particular differences (the *constituents* of Bertrand Russell, or the *ideas* of Plato): 'I can think of no better expression to characterise these similarities than "family resemblance"; for the various resemblances between members of a family – build, features, colour of eyes, gait, temperament, and so on and so forth – overlap and criss-cross in the same way.' Wittgenstein, *Philosophical Investigations*, §66–7.

43 These conditions constitute a *background* in the sense articulated by Taylor.

44 Wittgenstein, *Philosophical Investigations*, 241–2, emphasis in original.

45 In making this analogy Wittgenstein is not affirming that language is a method of measurement or that speaking is a sort of measuring. This analogy aims only to illustrate that language, as well as the practice of measurement, is ultimately grounded in a form of living activity, in a human *form of life*.

46 'You cannot use words to do what we do with them until you are initiate of the forms of life which give those words the point and shape they have in our lives.' Stanley

Cavell, 'Excursus on Wittgenstein's Vision of Language', in Crary and Read, *New Wittgenstein*, 33.

47 As Wittgenstein explicitly underlines, his philosophical approach should not be mistaken for pragmatism: 'But you aren't a pragmatist. No. For I am not saying that a proposition is true if it is useful. The usefulness, i.e. the use, gives the proposition its special sense, the language-game gives it.' Ludwig Wittgenstein, *Remarks on the Philosophy of Psychology, Volume 1*, trans. Gertrude E. M. Anscombe (London: Wiley-Blackwell, 1991), §266.

48 'What counts as an adequate test of a statement belongs to logic.' Wittgenstein, *Philosophical Investigations*, §82.

49

> But if someone were to say 'So logic too is an empirical science' he would be wrong. Yet this is right: the same proposition may get treated at one time as something to test by experience, at another as a rule of testing. [...] I want to say: propositions of the form of empirical propositions, and not only propositions of logic, form the foundation of all operating with thoughts (with language). (Wittgenstein, *Philosophical Investigations*, §98, §401)

50 Wittgenstein, *Philosophical Investigations*, §108.

51 Wittgenstein, *Philosophical Investigations*, emphasis in original.

52 'When Wittgenstein says "*Essence* is expressed by grammar" (§371), he is not denying the importance, or significance, of the concept of essence, but retrieving it. The need for essence is satisfied by grammar, if we see our real need.' Cavell, *Condition Handsome and Unhandsome*, 34.

53 Locke, *Essay Concerning Human Understanding*, book 3, chapter 2, section 8.

54 Wittgenstein, *Philosophical Investigations*, §293, emphasis in original.

55 Cora Diamond, 'Does Bismarck Have a Beetle in His Box? The Private Language Argument in the *Tractatus*', in *The New Wittgenstein*, ed. Alice Crary and Rupert Read (London: Routledge, 2000), 262–93.

56 'The private object is one about which neither he who has it nor he who hasn't got it can say anything to other or to himself.' Ludwig Wittgenstein, 'Notes for the Philosophical Lecture', in *Philosophical Occasions: 1912–1951* (Oxford: Hackett, 1993), 451.

57 Wittgenstein, 'Notes for the Philosophical Lecture', 275.

58 Cora Diamond, 'Does Bismarck have a Beetle in the Box?', in Crary and Read, *New Wittgenstein*, 274.

59 The instinctive tendency to understand things in a certain way is seen by Wittgenstein as connected to the fact that certain pictures are integrated in our language, and therefore in our lives. According to him, the validity of these pictures is strictly connected to the role that they have for the life of the people that incorporate them: depending on the particular case, pictures can be more or less adequate, more or less responsive to the needs of the agent or to the characteristics of the context:

> Let us suppose that our picture of thinking was a human being, leaning his head on his hand while he talks to himself. Our question is not 'Is that a correct picture?' but 'How is this picture employed as a picture of thinking?'. Say, not: 'We have formed a wrong picture of thinking' – but: 'We don't know our way about in the use of our picture, or of our pictures'. And hence we don't know our way about in the use of a word. (Wittgenstein, *Remarks on the Philosophy of Psychology*, §549)

60 I claim that this affirmation is 'misleading' and not 'mistaken' because it is not, in my view, completely wrong. Knowledge and language presuppose indeed a background, something that cannot be wholly articulated, and this implies that we always take something for granted when we speak and think. As Wittgenstein writes, 'It may be for example that *all enquiry on our part* is set so as to exempt certain propositions from doubt, if they are ever formulated. They lie apart from the route travelled by enquiry.' 'The *facts* of human natural history that throw light on our problem, are difficult for us to find out, for our talk passes them by, it is occupied with other things. (In the same way we tell someone: "Go into the shop and buy …" – not: "Put your left foot in front of your right foot etc. etc., then put coins down on the counter, etc. etc.")'. Bearing this in mind, we could speak of a 'direct' access to refer to the certainties that are at ground of our activities. However, this is not the way in which the idea of 'direct' access is generally used, and the idea of 'direct' knowledge is not necessary to proceed with my argument. For these reasons, I have chosen to stress the confusion generated by the term instead of underlining its potentialities. Wittgenstein, *On Certainty*, §88; Wittgenstein, *Remarks on the Philosophy of Psychology*, §78, emphasis in original.

61 By saying 'part of' I do not mean that they can be ideally separated by the background or that the background is a 'sum' of different things – the background works as a *whole*, and even if it can be articulated, its articulations cannot be ideally detached from it. By saying 'part of' I mean simply that the background is not constituted *only* by values and reasons.

62 Wittgenstein, *Philosophical Investigations*, §202, emphasis in original.

63 As I have underlined, the dialogical conception conceptualizes language as intrinsically open to mistake and does not guarantee the efficacy of particular instances of human understanding and communication. Language and knowledge are fallible, and there are always new and unexpected ways in which humans can commit epistemological mistakes, be misunderstood or fail to communicate.

64 Taylor, *Philosophical Arguments*, 13–15.

65 I could have said 'autonomy is constitutively dependent from a set of conditions *external* to the individual', but at this point of the argument I hope to have made clear that the distinction between internal and external conditions is generally deceptive in relation to the current debate on the concept of autonomy. What we call an 'individual' or an 'autonomous agent' is intrinsically embedded in a dialogical framework and therefore cannot be ideally detached from the context in which it occurs.

66 As we have seen, procedural and causally relational theories of autonomy belong to this group of perspectives. One of the most emblematic formulations of this view can be found in English Law regarding medical consent: '[The right of choice] exists notwithstanding that the reasons for making the choice are rational, irrational, unknown, or even non-existent'; *Re T (Adult: Refusal of Medical Treatment)* (1992).

67 Among the relational theorists analysed in this book, Oshana and Meyers explicitly analyse autonomy from a global point of view, while Benson and Christman defend a local approach to autonomy. Diana T. Meyers, 'Intersectional Identity and the Authentic Self? Opposite Attract', in Mackenzie and Stoljar, *Relational Autonomy*, 151–80; Oshana, 'Personal Autonomy and Society'; Benson, 'Taking Ownership'; Christman, 'Autonomy and Personal History'.

68 Benson, 'Taking Ownership', 120.

69 Christman, 'Autonomy and Personal History'.

70 The fact that this book is concerned with a specific case, however, does not imply that my argument is disconnected from other cases of problematic assessment of autonomy, but only that any problematic case requires a focus on the particulars that is structurally incompatible with an omnicomprehensive model of autonomy.

71 Christman, 'Autonomy and Personal History', 3.

72 Christman, 'Autonomy and Personal History'.

73 The dialogical conditions analysed in this chapter are not supposed to replace the entire set of procedural and functional conditions of autonomy (both regarding their theoretical role and their pragmatic application within particular legislations) but rather to integrate and refine them – where necessary.

74 As the discussion in Chapter 4 of constitutively and causally relational conceptions of autonomy implies, if self-worth is a condition of the *exercise* of autonomy, it is also a condition of its *development*.

75 See Chapter 3.

76 Benson, 'Free Agent and Self-Worth', 656–7.

77 Benson, 'Free Agent and Self-Worth', 650.

78 Mackenzie and Stoljar, *Relational Autonomy*, 140.

79 I follow Benson and Cudd in considering self-esteem a subcategory or a synonym of self-worth. However, given the relevance I have attributed to the concepts of 'worth' and 'importance' for the dialogical conception of the agent, I prefer using the term 'self-worth'. Benson, 'Free Agent and Self-Worth'; Cudd, *Analyzing Oppression*, 176–7.

80 Benson, 'Free Agent and Self-Worth', 659.

81 See Chapter 4.

82 I shall analyse in depth this question in the next chapter.

83 Robert S. Dillon, 'Toward a Feminist Conception of Self-Respect', *Hypatia* 7, no. 1 (1992): 52–69.

84 See Chapter 4.

85 Dillon, 'Toward a Feminist Conception of Self-Respect', 62.

86 Joel Anderson and Alex Honneth, 'Autonomy, Vulnerability, Recognition, and Justice', in *Autonomy and the Challenges to Liberalism: New Essays*, ed. John Christman and Joel Anderson (Cambridge: Cambridge University Press, 2009), 127–49.

87 Anderson and Honnet, 'Autonomy, Vulnerability, Recognition, and Justice', 62–3.

88 Govier, 'Self-Trust, Autonomy, and Self-Esteem'.

89 McLeod and Sherwin (2000); C. McLeod, *Self-Trust and Reproductive Autonomy* (Cambridge, MA: MIT Press, 2002).

90 McLeod, 'Relational Autonomy, Self-Trust and Health Care'.

91 McLeod, 'Relational Autonomy, Self-Trust and Health Care', 262–3.

92 In my view, these three conditions of self-trust should not be interpreted as independent from the other or as categorical distinctions, but as an analytical tool that can be helpful in identifying the variety of ways in which self-trust interacts with autonomy.

93 McLeod, 'Relational Autonomy, Self-Trust and Health Care', 263–4.

94 Govier, in contrast to McLeod, endorses a procedural and value-neutral approach to self-trust. Given that I have already underlined that procedural and 'radical' value-neutral accounts of autonomy generate contradictions, I shall dedicate more space to the analysis of McLeod's account instead of criticizing Govier's assumption about autonomy. See Govier, 'Self-Trust, Autonomy, and Self-Esteem'.

95 McLeod, *Self-Trust and Reproductive Autonomy*, 121–2.

96

> The agent can be given opportunities to develop and use her various capacities and, through these opportunities, learn to trust her capacities; the agent can receive encouragement from others to trust her own capacities. On the first level, the self-trust is relational in a causal sense; supportive social conditions provide the materials for its development. On the second level, self-trust is relational in a constitutive sense; the agent's trust in herself exists in part because others reinforce that trust in their relationships with her. (McLeod, *Self-Trust and Reproductive Autonomy*, 265)

97 Govier, 'Self-Trust, Autonomy, and Self-Esteem', 114–15.

98 McLeod, *Self-Trust and Reproductive Autonomy*, 104.

99 Westlund, 'Rethinking Relational Autonomy', 35.

100 Benson also underlines the relevance of dialogical answerability for autonomy; see Benson, 'Feminist Intuitions and the Normative Substance of Autonomy'; Paul Benson, 'Taking Ownership: Authority and Voice in Autonomous Agency', in *Autonomy and the Challenges to Liberalism: New Essays*, ed. John Christman and Joel Anderson (Cambridge: Cambridge University Press, 2009).

101 Benson's use of the adverb 'strangely' indicates, in my view, that his account is not fine-grained enough to adequately grasp the connection between dialogical answerability and autonomy. In my view, even if Benson's conception of autonomy is constitutively relational and weak substantivist, it does not take account of the dialogical constitution of knowledge and language, and therefore it cannot articulate completely why a lack of dialogical answerability can impair autonomy. Benson, 'Taking Ownership: Authority and Voice in Autonomous Agency', 34.

102 Benson, 'Taking Ownership: Authority and Voice in Autonomous Agency', 34.

103 Like Diana Meyers, Westlund affirms that her account is value-neutral despite its value-ladenness. As discussed in the first section of this chapter, the use of the label 'value-neutral' for value-laden, weakly substantive accounts, is fundamentally misleading. See also Paul Benson, 'Narrative Self-Understanding and Relational Autonomy: Comments on Catriona Mackenzie and Jacqui Poltera, "Narrative Integration, Fragmented Selves, and Autonomy" and Andrea C. Westlund "Rethinking Relational Autonomy"', *Symposia on Gender, Race and Philosophy* 7, no. 1 (2011): 1–5.

104 Martha Nussbaum, 'Political Liberalism and Respect: A Response to Linda Barclay', *SATS: Nordic Journal of Philosophy* 4, no. 2 (2003): 25–44.

105 Mackenzie, Rogers and Dodds, *Vulnerability*, 36.

106 The same reasoning applies to agents who want to become isolated and live in solitude; precisely because this choice or preference is made in radical contrast with the relational context, it is dialogically constituted.

107 Camillia Kong, *Mental Capacity in Relationship: Decision-Making, Dialogue, and Autonomy* (Cambridge: Cambridge University Press, 2017), 86–7.

108 Henrik Ibsen, *A Doll's House* (Wokingham: Dodo Press, 2005).

109 Cavell, *Condition Handsome and Unhandsome*, 109–11.

110 Cavell, *Condition Handsome and Unhandsome*, 112.

111 Nora says to Torvald that their last conversation 'is the first serious talk they have ever had, to which he replies, "Serious? What do you mean by that?"' Cavell, *Condition Handsome and Unhandsome*, 109.

112 Cavell, *Condition Handsome and Unhandsome*, 114.

113 We might suppose that, after Nora's departure, Torvald could have reflectively questioned the legitimacy of his judgements about his wife. Maybe he could also have overcome the distance that separated his view from Nora's, attaining a perspective, or a common horizon, in which Nora's claims are not seen as childish and silly, but as reasonable and worth articulating and actualizing. This process of dialogical enrichment – a process that Gadamer calls a 'fusion of horizon' – is the basis of the possibility of overcoming deep disagreements and the incompatibility of views such as those dividing Nora and Torvald: Hans-George Gadamer, *Truth and Method* (London: Bloomsbury, 1998), 317.

114 Mackenzie, Rogers and Dodds, *Vulnerability*, 38.

Chapter 6

1 For a detailed analysis of this question and of its implications, see Chapter 2.

2 For a defence of the approach adopted by judges to anorexia see Eric C. Ip, 'Anorexia Nervosa, Advance Directives, and the Law: A British Perspective', *Bioethics* 33, no. 8 (2019): 931–6.

3 Martha A. Fineman, 'The Vulnerable Subject and the Responsive State', *Emory Law Journal* 60, no. 2 (2010): 251–75.

4 The MCA does not offer a definition of best interests; it only asserts that 'an act done, or decision made, under this Act for or on behalf of a person who lacks capacity must be done, or made, in his best interests'. However, as Wayne Martin and colleagues have argued, the courts have interpreted the practice of best interest decisions in an individualistic manner. The Public Guardian articulates the idea of best interest decisions in this way: 'Anything done for a person who cannot make decisions for themselves must be in their best interests. This means thinking about what is best for the person, and not about what anyone else wants.' The Mental Health Foundation explains it in a similar manner: 'When decisions are made for someone they must be made in their best interests. This means that what is decided must be best for that person and not what someone else wants.' Wayne Martin, Fabian Freyenhagen, Elizabeth Hall, Tom O'Shea, Antal Szerletics and Vivienne Ashley, 'An Unblinkered View of Best Interests', *BMJ* (Online) (2012); Andrew Holman and Steph Moore, *Making Decisions: An Easyread Guide*, 2nd edn (London: Office of the Public Guardian, 2007); Mental Health Foundation, *Banking on Good Decisions: How Can the Mental Capacity Act Help You with Your Bank, Building Society or Post Office Account?* (London: Mental Health Foundation, 2008).

5 Sullivan and Niker, 'Relational Autonomy, Paternalism, and Maternalism', 656, emphasis added.

6 Denise Kästner, Bernd Löwe and Antje Gumz, 'The Role of Self-Esteem in the Treatment of Patients with Anorexia Nervosa – a Systematic Review and Meta-Analysis', *International Journal of Eating Disorders* 52, no. 2 (2019): 101–16.

7 Kästner, Löwe and Gumz, 'The Role of Self-Esteem', 102.

8 Brytek-Matera, 'Anorexia Nervosa among French Adolescent', 53.

9 Romin W. Tafarodi and William B. Swann Jr, 'Self-Liking and Self-Competence as Dimensions of Global Self-Esteem: Initial Validation of a Measure', *Journal of Personality Assessment* 65, no. 2 (2010): 322–42.

10 Tafarodi and Swann, 'Self-Liking and Self-Competence', 325.

11 Tafarodi and Swann, 'Self-Liking and Self-Competence', emphasis added.

12 Benson, 'Free Agent and Self-Worth', 650.

13 Jamie-Lee Pennesi and Tracey D. Wade, 'A Systematic Review of the Existing Models of Disordered Eating: Do They Inform the Development of Effective Interventions?', *Clinical Psychology Review* 43 (2016): 175–92; Anna Oldershaw, Helen Startup and Tony Lavander, 'Anorexia Nervosa and a Lost Emotional Self: A Psychological Formulation of the Development, Maintenance, and Treatment of Anorexia Nervosa', *Frontiers in Psychology* 10, no. 219 (2019): 1–22; Anna Brytek-Matera, 'Anorexia Nervosa among French Adolescent Females in Relation to Self-Esteem, Coping Strategies, Anger Expression and Anger Control', *Archives of Psychiatry and Psychotherapy* 4 (2007): 53–7; Ewa Karpowicz, Ingela Skärsäter and Lauri Nevonen, 'Self-Esteem in Patients Treated for Anorexia Nervosa', *International Journal of Mental Health Nursing* 18, no. 5 (2009): 318–25; Kästner, Löwe and Gumz, 'The Role of Self-Esteem'.

14 Cristopher G. Fairburn, Zafra Cooper and Roz Shafran, 'Cognitive Behaviour Therapy for Eating Disorders: A "Transdiagnostic" Theory and Treatment', *Behaviour Research and Therapy* 41, no. 5 (2003): 509–28.

15 Timo Brockmeyer, Martin G. Holtforth, Hinrich Bents, Annette Kämmerer, Wolfgang Herzog and Hans-Christoph Friederich, 'The Thinner the Better: Self-Esteem and Low Body Weight in Anorexia Nervosa', *Clinical Psychology and Psychotherapy* 20, no. 5 (2013): 294–300.

16 This characterization applies chiefly to those anorexics who have never received psychological treatment or who are in the early and acute phase of the disorder; Brockmeyer, Holtforth, Bents, Kämmerer, Herzog and Friederich, 'The Thinner the Better'.

17 Theroux, 'Talking to Anorexia', emphasis in original.

18 Theroux, 'Talking to Anorexia'; Anna Oldershaw, Helen Startup and Tony Lavender, 'Anorexia and a Lost Emotional Self'; Henning Schauenburg, Hans-Cristoph Friederich, Beate Wild and Stephan Zipfel, 'Focal Psychodynamic Psychotherapy of Anorexia Nervosa: A Treatment Manual', *Psychotherapeut* 54, no. 4 (2009): 270–80.

19 Amy M. Lampard, Giorgio A. Tasca, Louise Balfour and Hany Bissada, 'An Evaluation of the Transdiagnostic Cognitive-Behavioural Model of Eating Disorders', *European Eating Disorders Review* 21, no. 2 (2013): 99–107.

20 Brockmeyer, Holtforth, Bents, Kämmerer, Herzog and Friederich, 'The Thinner the Better'.

21 Inger Halvorsen and Sonja Heyerdahl, 'Girls with Anorexia Nervosa as Young Adults: Personality, Self-Esteem, and Life Satisfaction', *International Journal of Eating Disorders* 39, no. 4 (2006): 285–93; Brockmeyer, Holtforth, Bents, Kämmerer, Herzog and Friederich, 'The Thinner the Better'.

22 Tan, Hope, Stewart and Fitzpatrick, 'Competence to Make Treatment Decisions in Anorexia'.

23 Claudine Clucas, 'Understanding Self-Respect and Its Relationship to Self-Esteem', *Personality and Social Psychology Bulletin* 46, no. 6 (2020): 855.

24 Hope, Tan, Stewart and Fitzpatrick, 'Anorexia Nervosa and the Language of Authenticity'; Conti, 'Recovering Identity from Anorexia Nervosa'.

25 Norris, Gleaves and Hutchinson, 'Anorexia Nervosa and Perfectionism'.

26 Dillon, 'Toward a Feminist Conception of Self-Respect'.

27 Dillon, 'Toward a Feminist Conception of Self-Respect', 263–4.

28 Tan, Hope, Stewart and Fitzpatrick, 'Control and Compulsory Treatment in Anorexia'.

29 Special Books by Special Kids, 'Battling Chronic Anorexia for Over a Decade'.

30 Tan, Hope and Stewart, 'Competence to Refuse Treatment in Anorexia'.

31 Hope, Tan, Stewart and McMillan, 'Agency, Ambivalence and Authenticity'.

32 Tan, Hope, Stewart and Fitzpatrick, 'Competence to Make Treatment Decisions in Anorexia'.

33 Govier, 'Self-Trust, Autonomy, and Self-Esteem'.

34 Hope, Tan, Stewart and McMillan, 'Agency, Ambivalence and Authenticity'.

35 Hope, Tan, Stewart and McMillan, 'Agency, Ambivalence and Authenticity'.

36 Hope, Tan, Stewart and Fitzpatrick, 'Anorexia Nervosa and the Language of Authenticity'.

37 Hope, Tan, Stewart and Fitzpatrick, 'Anorexia Nervosa and the Language of Authenticity'.

38

> Engaging directly with the decision maker in the ways advocated here may be very difficult. People at the severe end of the illness may be very medically unwell, and too weak to attend a hearing, complicating the court's ability to directly question the adult. It also may be difficult for the person whose capacity is questioned to be directly confronted with what the court sees as their distortions

of reality. Nevertheless, despite these difficulties, direct and open engagement with the adult on the issue of capacity is essential for proper decision making. Without it, for people with anorexia who are refusing treatment, there is a serious ongoing risk of their capacity being decided on their diagnosis alone, something capacity law is supposed to avoid. Moreover, without this engagement, authorised invasion of the subjects' bodily integrity may occur without their having any voice in the process. (Sam Boyle, 'How Should the Law Determine Capacity to Refuse Treatment for Anorexia?', *International Journal of Law and Psychiatry* 64 (2019): 257)

39 As Camillia Kong underlines, judges usually overturn clinicians' judgement about anorexics' decisional capacity. As I shall argue, dialogical answerability cannot be assessed from a univocal point of view, and it requires the participation of clinicians and patients' significant others. Camillia Kong, 'Beyond the Balancing Scales: The Importance of Prejudice and Dialogue in *A Local Authority v E et al.*', *Child and Family Law Quarterly* 26, no. 2 (2014): 216–36.

40 There's also in fact a third possibility: the assessors might make a mistake in the assessment of the patient's dialogical answerability. I shall take into account this case when I deal with the variety of circumstances in which the dialogical assessment can turn out to be oppressive for the patient.

41 Michel Foucault, *The Birth of the Clinic: An Archaeology of Medical Perception*, trans. Alan M. Sheridan (London: Routledge, 2003).

42 Andrea LaMarre, Michael P. Levine, Su Holmes and Helen Malson, 'An Open Invitation to Productive Conversations about Feminism and the Spectrum of Eating Disorders (Part 1): Basic Principles of Feminist Approaches', *Journal of Eating Disorders* 10, no. 54 (2022): 1–12; Sacha K. Jamieson, Jacinta Tan, Kym Piekunka, Shannon Calvert and Stephen Anderson, 'Navigating the Ethical Complexities of Severe and Enduring Eating Disorders: Tools for Critically Reflective Practice and Collaborative Decision-Making', *Journal of Eating Disorders* 12, no. 134 (2024): 1–17.

43 Kate Young, Jane Fisher and Maggie Kirkman, '"Do Mad People Get Endo or Does Endo Make You Mad?": Clinicians' Discoursive Construction of Medicine and Women with Endometriosis', *Feminism & Psychology* 29, no. 3 (2019): 337–56; Deborah Lupton, *Medicine as Culture: Illness, Disease, and the Body* (Thousand Oaks, CA: Sage Books, 2012).

44 Anti-oppression trainings should be able to deliver an elementary knowledge of the main questions connected to oppression, such as intersectionality, power and privilege, as well as to provide basic tools for the recognition and handling of these factors. Crucially, in order to offer a body of knowledge useful from the practical aims of the assessment, the training must include data about the peculiar kind of oppression experienced by the patient as a patient and as intersectional situated subject. In this regard, considered that this knowledge comes in part from the experience of oppressed groups and individual, it is necessary to involve them in the structurization of anti-oppression trainings.

45 Kong, *Mental Capacity in Relationship*, 232.

46 Taylor underlines that the exercise of practical reasoning in cases of moral disagreement does not imply that we have 'to convince those who are dividedly and unconfusedly attached to one first principle that they ought to shift to an entirely different one … Rather, we are always trying to show that, granted what our interlocutors already accept, they cannot but attribute to the acts or policies in dispute the significance we are urging.' Taylor, *Philosophical Arguments*, 42.

47 Serene Khader, 'Beyond Autonomy Fetishism: Affiliation with Autonomy in Women's Empowerment', *Journal of Human Development and Capabilities* 17, no. 1 (2016): 130.

48 In a more recent article, Giordano has argued that 'the exceptional circumstances that characterize anorexia justify a partial derogation from the principle of respect for autonomy'. I disagree with this approach, first, because it recommends the same kind of mistake that it aims to solve and, second, because it impedes the articulation of the problems raised by anorexia with regard to the concept of autonomy. There is no need to adopt exceptionalism as a principle of ethical decision-making regarding anorexia; Giordano, 'A Case for Exceptionalism', 321–2.

49 Keel, 'Update on Course and Outcome in Eating Disorders'.

50 Pro-ana websites and communities typically describe anorexic self-control as a superior good.

51 The relation between anorexia and religious or spiritual commitment has been addressed in detail. What I want to stress here is that, even admitting the analogy between anorexic and religious or spiritual commitments, there are no sufficient reasons to acknowledge the agent's decisional capacity on the sole ground of their assertions about their hypergoods and metaphysical beliefs. An agent who is dialogically answerable must be able to articulate their commitment to their values in an intelligible way. It is not, as Nussbaum claims, that the assessment of dialogical answerability is *intrinsically* incompatible with religious commitments. As Mackenzie argues, the assessment of dialogical answerability is not 'inconsistent per se with religious commitment, but it is inconsistent with dogmatic forms of religious commitment, or any other form of dogmatism, for that matter, which involve appeals to authority that bypass a person's reflective agency': Mackenzie, Rogers and Dodds, *Vulnerability*, 36; Nussbaum, 'Political Liberalism and Respect'. See also Emma White, *The Spirituality of Anorexia: A Goddess Feminist Theology* (London: Routledge, 2018); Alexandra Pittock, 'How Are Anorexia Nervosa and Spirituality Connected, and What Implications Does This Have for Treatment?', *Royal College of Psychiatrists* 1 (2014): 1–14; Forcen, 'Anorexia Mirabilis'; Weinberg, 'From the Ascetic Ideal to the Esthetic Ideal'; Pearce, 'Richard Morton'; Joan M. Griffin and Elliot M. Berry, 'A Modern Day Holy Anorexia? Religious Language in Advertising and Anorexia Nervosa in the West', *European Journal of Clinical Nutrition* 57 (2003): 43–51; Helen Baxter, 'Religion and Eating Disorder', *European Eating Disorders Review* 9 (2001): 137–9; Sarah Huline-Dickens, 'Anorexia Nervosa: Some Connections with the Religious Attitude', *British Journal of Medical Psychology* 73, no. 1 (2000): 67–76.

52 Strife and Rickard, 'The Conceptualization of Anorexia'.

53 Almost every pro-ana website I have visited reports a version of the so-called *Ana Commandments*:

> 1) If you aren't thin you aren't attractive; 2) being thin is more important than being healthy; 3) you must buy smaller clothes, cut your hair, take diet pills, starve yourself, do anything to make yourself look thinner; 4) thou shall not eat without feeling guilty; 5) thou shall not eat fattening food without punishing oneself afterwards; 6) thou shall count calories and restrict intake accordingly; 7) what the scale says is the most important thing; 8) losing weight is good / gaining weight is bad; 9) you can never be too thin; 10) being thin and not eating are signs of true will power and success.

Like the ten commandments of the Judeo-Christian tradition, these commandments represent the basic principles that regulate the life of the '*good* anorexic', or, in the terms by pro-ana users, of the 'devotee to Ana' (the 'divine' personification of anorexia, 'often portrayed as a sort of deity, someone to be obeyed at all costs, requiring complete sacrifice of appetite and personal wishes').

54 Relations are generally described by pro-ana users as an impediment for the attaining and maintenance of anorexic self-control, and pro-ana websites have plenty of pages about advices on hiding anorexia from friends and family. Yet, the value and role pro-ana users attribute to relation with others is often ambivalent. On the one hand, such relations are considered detrimental to the 'real' concerns and commitments of pro-ana users, while, on the other hand, they constitute a constant and fundamental background for the social recognition of their anorexic self-control, will-power and self-worth.

55 Tan, Hope, Stewart and Fitzpatrick, 'Competence to Make Treatment Decisions in Anorexia'.

56 Hope, Tan, Stewart and McMillan, 'Agency, Ambivalence and Authenticity'.

57 Hope, Tan, Stewart and Fitzpatrick, 'Anorexia Nervosa and the Language of Authenticity'.

58 Colleen Schreyer, Janelle W Coughlin, Saniha H Makhzoumi, Graham W. Redgrave, Jennifer L. Hansen and Angela S. Guarda, 'Perceived Coercion in Inpatients with Anorexia Nervosa: Associations with Illness Severity and Hospital Course', *International Journal of Eating Disorders* 49, no. 4 (2016): 407–12.

59 Anne Ward, Rosalind Ramsay, Gerald Russell and Janet Treasure, 'Follow-Up Mortality Study of Compulsorily Treated Patients with Anorexia Nervosa', *International Journal of Eating Disorders* 48, no. 7 (2015): 860–5.

60 The term 'severe and enduring' has typically been used to designate mental disorders that include psychosis among their symptoms, but in recent years it has also been applied to eating disorders. Phillipa Hay and Stephen Touyz, 'Treatment of Patients with Severe and Enduring Eating Disorders', *Current Opinion in Psychiatry* 28, no. 6 (2015): 473–7.

61 American Psychiatric Association, DSM-V.

62 Department of Health and Social Care, *National Service Framework for Mental Health* (London: Department of Health and Social Care, 1999), 43

63 Paul Robinson, *Severe and Enduring Eating Disorder (SEED). Management of Complex Presentations of Anorexia and Bulimia Nervosa* (New Jersey: Wiley-Blackwell, 2009), 8.

64 Catherine C. Broomfield, Kristin Stedal, Stephen Touyz and Paul Rhodes, 'Labeling and Defining Severe and Enduring Anorexia Nervosa: A Systematic Review and Critical Analysis', *International Journal of Eating Disorders* 50, no. 6 (2017): 611–23.

65 Phillipa Hay and Stephen Touyz, 'Classification Challenges in the Field of Eating Disorders: Can Severe and Enduring Anorexia Nervosa Be Better Defined?', *Journal of Eating Disorders* 6, no. 41 (2018): 1–3; Phillipa Hay and Stephen Touyz, 'Treatment for Severe and Enduring Anorexia Nervosa: A Review', *Australian and New Zealand Journal of Psychiatry* 46, no. 12 (2012): 1136–44; Stephen Touyz, Daniel Le Grange, Hubert J. Lacey and Phillipa Hay, eds, *Managing Severe and Enduring Anorexia Nervosa: A Clinician's Guide* (London: Taylor and Francis, 2016).

66 I am assuming that the patient has already undergone the standard therapies for anorexia: family-based therapy and cognitive behavioural therapy.

67 Arcelus, 'Mortality Rates in Patients with Anorexia'.

68 Emma Cave and Jacinta Tan, 'Severe and Enduring Anorexia Nervosa in the Court of Protection in England and Wales', *International Journal of Mental Health and Capacity Law* 23, no. 17 (2017): 4–24.

69 Robinson, *Severe and Enduring Eating Disorder*, 6.

70 June Alexander, 'Severe and Enduring Anorexia Nervosa – Should We Even Give Up?', *Diary Healer*, Web Blog, https://www.thediaryhealer.com/2017/09/12/severe-and-enduring-anorexia-nervosa-should-we-ever-give-up (accessed 18 April 2019).

71 Stephen Touyz and Phillipa Hay, 'Severe and Enduring Anorexia Nervosa (SEAN): In Search of a New Paradigm', *Journal of Eating Disorders* 3, no. 26 (2015): 1–3.

72 Zipfel, Giel, Bulik, Hay and Schmidt, 'Aetiology, Assessment and Treatment'.

73 Deep Brain Stimulation is a surgical procedure involving the placement of an electrical stimulator in the brain. The stimulator sends electrical impulses to specific targets to change the activity of the brain.

74 Rebecca J. Park, Ilina Singh, Alexandra C. Pike and Jacinta O. Tan, 'Deep Brain Stimulation in Anorexia Nervosa: Hope for the Hopeless or Exploitation of the Vulnerable? The Oxford Neuroethics Gold Standard Framework', *Frontiers in Psychiatry* 8, no. 44 (2017): 1–10.

75 Giordano, 'A Case for Exceptionalism', 326.

76 In some circumstances, SEAN has been considered terminal. But the entire symptomatology of anorexia remains reversible – especially if compared with other terminal stages of diseases such as lung cancer, leukaemia or Lesch-Nyhan syndrome. See Cave and Tan, 'Severe and Enduring Anorexia Nervosa'; Samantha Schmidt S., 'Anorexic Woman Weighing 69 Pounds Has a Right to Starve, Court Rules', *Washington Post*, 22 November 2016, https://www.washingtonpost.com/gdpr-consent/?next_url=https%3a%2f%2fwww.washingtonpost.com%2fnews%2fmorning-mix%2fwp%2f2016%2f11%2f22%2fanorexic-woman-weighing-69-pounds-has-a-right-to-starve-court-rules%2f (accessed 22 December 2018).

77 Giordano, 'A Case for Exceptionalism', 316, 326.

78 Giordano, 'A Case for Exceptionalism', 327.

79 Janet Conti, Paul Rhodes and Heather Adams, 'Listening in the Dark: Why We Need Stories of People Living with Severe and Enduring Anorexia Nervosa', *Journal of Eating Disorders* 4, no. 33 (2016): 1–7.

80 Riccardo Dalla Grave, Marwan El Ghoch, Massimiliano Sartirana and Simona Calugi, 'Cognitive Behavioral Therapy for Anorexia Nervosa: An Update', *Current Psychiatry Reports* 18, no. 1 (2016): 1–18.

81 Almut Zeeck, Beate Herpertz-Dahlmann, Hans-Christoph Friederich, Timo Brockmeyer, Gaby Resmark, Ulrich Hagenah, Stefan Ehrlich, Ulrich Cuntz, Stephan Zipfel and Armin Hartmann, 'Psychotherapeutic Treatment for Anorexia Nervosa: A Systematic Review and Network Meta-Analysis', *Frontiers in Psychiatry* 9, no. 158 (2018): 1–14.

82 Paul H. Robinson, Roza Kukucska, Giulia Guidetti and Gerard Leavey, 'Severe and Enduring Anorexia Nervosa (SEED-AN): A Qualitative Study of Patients with 20+ Years of Anorexia Nervosa', *European Eating Disorders Review* 23, no. 4 (2015): 320.

83 Giordano, 'A Case for Exceptionalism'.

84 Freddy Burke, Maree Higgins and Maureen MacGinley, '"I'll Do It on My Own, but I'm Never Alone": Lived Experience and Practitioner Perspectives of Autonomy in Longstanding and Severe Eating Disorder Treatment and Recovery – a Rapid Evidence Review', *Journal of Eating Disorders* 12, no. 208 (2024): 402–23.

85 Royal College of Psychiatrists, *PS03/19 Position Statement on Early Intervention for Eating Disorders* (London: Royal College of Psychiatrists, 2019); Paul Rodhe, Eric Stice and Nathan C. Marti, 'Development and Predictive Effects of Eating Disorder Risk Factors during Adolescence: Implications for Prevention Efforts', *International Journal of Eating Disorders* 48, no. 2 (2015): 187–98.

Conclusion

1 More precisely, the presence of such private factors together with a functioning set of procedural capacities is not sufficient to infer the mental capacity of the agent.

2 A very interesting alternative perspective on the relation between liberalism, individualism and feminism is offered by Lisa Downing, *Selfish Women* (London: Routledge, 2019).

3 My study of autonomy and anorexia has allowed me to individuate these four conditions, but further research in other domains is required to gain a wider understanding of the conditions for the exercise of autonomy. For example, previous studies of the Essex Autonomy Project about the capacity to refuse treatment for patients with affective disorder have found that 'in both severe depression and mania, the future can be experienced in a radically anomalous way which can undermine decision making capacity for treatment'. Gareth S. Owen, Wayne Martin and Tania Gergel, 'Misevaluating the Future: Affective Disorder and Decision-Making Capacity for Treatment – a Temporal Understanding', *Psychopathology* 51, no. 6 (2018): 371–9.

4 Tafarodi and Swann, 'Self-Liking and Self-Competence'.

Bibliography

Books

American Psychiatric Association. *Diagnostic and Statistical Manual of Mental Disorders: Diagnostic and Statistical Manual of Mental Disorders*, 5th edn. Arlington: American Psychiatric Association, 2013.
Anderson, Joel, and Christman, John, eds. *Autonomy and the Challenges to Liberalism: New Essays*. Cambridge: Cambridge University Press, 2005.
Anthony, Louise. M., and Witt, Charlotte E., eds. *A Mind of One's Own: Feminist Essays on Reason and Objectivity*. London: Routledge, 2002.
Augustine. *Confessions*. Translated by Henry Chadwick. Oxford: Oxford University Press, 1998.
Ball, Terence, James, Farr, and Russell, Hanson L., eds. *Political Innovation and Conceptual Change*. Cambridge: Cambridge University Press, 1989.
Bateson, Gregory. *Steps to an Ecology of Mind*. Chicago: University of Chicago Press, 1972.
Berlin, Isaiah. *Liberty: Incorporating Four Essays on Liberty*. Oxford: Oxford University Press, 2002.
Bordo, Susan, *Unbearable Weight: Feminism, Western Culture, and the Body*. Berkeley: University of California Press, 1993.
Brandom, Robert B. *Making It Explicit*. Cambridge: Harvard University Press, 1998.
Brecher, Robert. *Getting What You Want? A Critique of Liberal Morality*. London: Routledge, 1997.
Brownell, Kelly D., and Fairburn, Cristopher G., eds. *Eating Disorders and Obesity: A Comprehensive Handbook*. New York: Guilford Press, 1995.
Bruch, Hilde. *Eating Disorders: Obesity, Anorexia Nervosa and the Person Within*. London: Routledge and Kegan Paul, 1974.
Burkert, Nathalie T. *Psychological and Neurobiological Aspects of Eating Disorders. A Taste-fMRI Study in Patients Suffering from Anorexia Nervosa*. New York: Springer, 2016.
Cavell, Stanley. *Condition Handsome and Unhandsome: The Constitution of Emersonian Perfectionism. The Carus Lectures 1988*. Chicago: University of Chicago Press, 1990.
Christman, John. *The Politics of Persons. Individual Autonomy and Socio-Historical Selves*. Cambridge: Cambridge University Press, 2009.
Code, Lorraine. *What Can She Know? Feminist Theory and the Construction of Knowledge*. New York: Cornell University Press, 1991.
Condillac, Étienne B. *Essay on the Origin of Human Knowledge*. Cambridge: Cambridge University Press, 2001.
Conly, Sarah. *Against Autonomy: Justifying Coercive Paternalism*. Cambridge: Cambridge University Press, 2013.

Crary, Alice, and Read, Rupert, eds. *The New Wittgenstein*. London: Routledge, 2000.
Cudd, Ann. *Analyzing Oppression*. Oxford: Oxford University Press, 2006.
Department for Constitutional Affairs. *Mental Capacity Act 2005: Code of Practice*. London: TSO, 2007.
Department of Health and Social Care. *National Service Framework for Mental Health*. London: Department of Health and Social Care, 1999.
Department of Health and Welsh Office. *Code of Practice: Mental Health Act 1983*. London: Stationery Office, 1999.
Descartes, René. *Discourse on Method and Meditations on First Philosophy*. Translated by Donald A. Cress. Indianapolis: Hackett, 1998.
Downing, Lisa. *Selfish Women*. London: Routledge, 2019.
Duker, Marilyn, and Slade, Roger. *Anorexia and Bulimia: How to Help*. Buckingham: Open University Press, 2003.
Elster, Jon. *Sour Grapes: Studies in the Subversion of Rationality*. Cambridge: Cambridge University Press, 1983.
Foucault, Michel. *The Birth of the Clinic: An Archaeology of Medical Perception*. Translated Alan M. Sheridan. London: Routledge, 2003.
Friedman, Marilyn. *Autonomy, Gender, Politics*. Oxford: Oxford University Press, 2003.
Gadamer, Hans G. *Truth and Method*. London: Bloomsbury, 1998.
Giordano, Simona. *Understanding Eating Disorders. Conceptual and Ethical Issues in the Treatment of Anorexia and Bulimia Nervosa*. Oxford: Oxford University Press, 2005.
Gutmann, Emy, ed. *Multiculturalism: Examining the Politics of Recognition*. Princeton: Princeton University Press, 1994).
Herder, Johann G. *On the Origin of Language*. Translated by John H. Moran and Alexander Gode. Chicago: University of Chicago Press, 1986.
Hobbes, Thomas. *Leviathan*. Oxford: Blackwell, 1989.
Holman, Andrew, and Moore, Steph. *Making Decisions: An Easyread Guide*, 2nd edn. London: Office of the Public Guardian, 2007.
Hume, David. *A Treatise of Human Nature by David Hume*, reprinted from the original edition in three volumes and edited, with an analytical index, by L. A. Selby-Bigge, MA. Oxford: Oxford University Press, 2018.
Hutchison, Katrina, Mackenzie, Catriona, and Marina, Oshana, eds. *Social Dimensions of Moral Responsibility*. Oxford: Oxford University Press, 2018.
Ibsen, Henrik. *A Doll's House*. Wokingham: Dodo Press, 2005.
Jaggar, Alison M. *Feminist Politics and Human Nature*. Totowa: Rowman & Allanhead, 1983.
Kant, Immanuel. *Lectures on Ethics*. Translated by Louis Infield. New York: Harper & Row, 1963.
Kant, Immanuel. *Grounding for the Metaphysics of Morals*. Translated by Mary Gregor. Indianapolis: Hackett, 1981.
Khader, Serene J. *Adaptive Preferences and Women's Empowerment*. Oxford: Oxford University Press, 2011.
Kong, Camillia. *Mental Capacity in Relationship: Decision-Making, Dialogue, and Autonomy*. Cambridge: Cambridge University Press, 2017.
Konner, Melvin. *The Evolution of Childhood*. Cambridge: Harvard University Press, 2010.
Laing, Ronald D., and Esterson, Aaron. *Sanity, Madness, and the Family*. London: Penguin Books, 1964.
Lemberg, Raymond. *Eating Disorders – a Reference Sourcebook*. Phoenix: Oryx Press, 1999.

Levin, Michael. *Feminism and Freedom*. New Brunswick: Transaction Books, 1987.
Locke, John. *An Essay Concerning Human Understanding*. London: Penguin Books, 1998.
Locke, John. *The Second Treatise on Civil Government*. Yale: Yale University Press, 2003.
Luker, Kristin. *Taking Choices: Abortion and the Decision Not to Contracept*. Berkeley: University of California Press, 1975.
Lupton, Deborah. *Medicine as Culture: Illness, Disease, and the Body*. Thousand Oaks: Sage Books, 2012.
MacIntyre, Alasdair. *After Virtue*. Notre Dame: University of Notre Dame Press, 1988.
MacIntyre, Alasdair. *Dependent Rational Animals: Why Human Beings Need the Virtues*. Chicago: Open Court, 1999.
Mackenzie, Catriona, Rogers, Wendy, and Dodds, Susan, eds. *Vulnerability: New Essays in Ethics and Feminist Philosophy*. Oxford: Oxford University Press, 2014.
Mackenzie, Catriona, and Stoljar, Natalie, eds. *Relational Autonomy: Feminist Perspectives on Autonomy, Agency, and the Social Self*. Oxford: Oxford University Press, 2000.
Macpherson, Crawford B. *The Political Theory of Possessive Individualism*. Oxford: Oxford University Press, 1962.
Marston, Greg, Jeremy, Moss, and Quiggin, John, eds. *Risk, Welfare and Work*. Melbourne: Melbourne University Press, 2010.
McLeod, Carolyn. *Self-Trust and Reproductive Autonomy*. Cambridge, MA: MIT Press, 2002.
Mead, George H. *Mind, Self and Society*. Chicago: University of Chicago Press, 1934.
Mele, Alfred. *Autonomous Agents: From Self-Control to Autonomy*. Oxford: Oxford University Press, 1995.
Mental Health Foundation. *Banking on Good Decisions: How Can the Mental Capacity Act Help You with Your Bank, Building Society or Post Office Account?* London: Mental Health Foundation, 2008.
Nussbaum, Martha. *Hiding from Humanity: Disgust, Shame, and the Law*. Princeton: Princeton University Press, 2004.
Oshana, Marina. *Personal Autonomy and Social Oppression*. New York: Routledge, 2015.
Palazzoli, Maria S., Cirillo, Stefano, Selvini, Matteo, and Sorrentino, Anna M. *Ragazze Anoressiche E Bulimiche: La Terapia Familiare*. Milan: Cortina, 1998.
Panksepp, Jaan, and Biven, Lucy. *The Archaeology of Mind: Neuroevolutionary Origins of Human Emotions*. London: W.W. Norton, 2012.
Quine, Willard V. 'Epistemology Naturalized'. *Ontological Relativity and Other Essays*. New York: Columbia University Press, 1969.
Robinson, Paul. *Severe and Enduring Eating Disorder (SEED). Management of Complex Presentations of Anorexia and Bulimia Nervosa*. New Jersey: Wiley-Blackwell, 2009.
Rorty, Richard. *Philosophy and the Mirror of Nature*. Princeton: Princeton University Press, 1979.
Royal College of Psychiatrists and Royal College of Physicians. *MARSIPAN: Management of Really Sick Patients with Anorexia Nervosa*, 2nd edn. London: College Report CR189, 2014.
Royal College of Psychiatrists. *PS03/19 Position Statement on Early Intervention for Eating Disorders*. London: Royal College of Psychiatrists, 2019.
Saukko, Paula. *The Anorexic Self. A Personal, Political Analysis of a Diagnostic Discourse*. New York: State University of New York, 2008.
Saussure, Ferdinand. *Course in General Linguistics*. New York: Philosophical Library, 1959.
Sen, Amartya K. *Development as Freedom*. Oxford: Oxford University Press, 1999.
Sen, Amartya K. *The Idea of Justice*. London: Penguin, 2010.

Silver, Anna K. *Victorian Literature and the Anorexic Body*. Cambridge: Cambridge University Press, 2002.
Taylor, Charles. *Philosophical Papers 1: Human Agency and Language*. Cambridge: Cambridge University Press, 1985.
Taylor, Charles. *Philosophical Papers 2: Philosophy and the Human Sciences*. Cambridge: Cambridge University Press, 1985.
Taylor, Charles. *Sources of Self. The Making of the Modern Identity*. Harvard: Harvard University Press, 1989.
Taylor, Charles. *The Ethics of Authenticity*. Harvard: Harvard University Press, 1991.
Taylor, Charles. *Multiculturalism. Examining the Politics of Recognition*. Princeton: Princeton University Press, 1994.
Taylor, Charles. *Philosophical Arguments*. Cambridge: Harvard University Press, 1995.
Taylor, Charles. *A Secular Age*. Cambridge: Harvard University Press, 2007.
Taylor, Charles. *Dilemmas and Connections*. Cambridge: Harvard University Press, 2011.
Taylor, Charles, and Dreyfus, Hubert. *Retrieving Realism*. Cambridge: Harvard University Press, 2015.
Taylor, Charles. *The Language Animal: The Full Shape of Human Linguistic Capacity*. Cambridge: Harvard University Press, 2016.
Taylor, James S. *Personal Autonomy: New Essays on Personal Autonomy and Its Role in Contemporary Moral Philosophy*. Cambridge: Cambridge University Press, 2005.
Todes, Samuel. *Body and World*. Cambridge: MIT Press, 2001.
Tomasello, Michael. *Origins of Human Communication*. Cambridge: MIT Press, 2008.
Tomasello, Michael. *Becoming Human: A Theory of Ontogeny*. Cambridge: Harvard University Press, 2019.
Touyz, Stephen, Le Grange, Daniel, Lacey, Hubert J., and Phillipa, Hay, eds. *Managing Severe and Enduring Anorexia Nervosa: A Clinician's Guide*. London: Taylor and Francis, 2016.
Veltman, Andrea, and Piper, Mark, eds. *Autonomy, Oppression, and Gender*. Oxford: Oxford University Press, 2014.
White, Emma. *The Spirituality of Anorexia. A Goddess Feminist Theology*. London: Routledge, 2018.
Williams, Bernard. *Moral Luck: Philosophical Papers 1973–1980*. Cambridge: Cambridge University Press, 1981.
Williams, Bernard. *Making Sense of Humanity: And Other Philosophical Papers 1982–1993*. Cambridge: Cambridge University Press, 1995.
Wittgenstein, Ludwig. *On Certainty*. Translated by Denis Paul and Gertrude E. M. Anscombe. Oxford: Basil Blackwell, 1969.
Wittgenstein, Ludwig. *Remarks on the Philosophy of Psychology P. 1*. Translated by Gertrude E. M. Anscombe. London: Wiley-Blackwell, 1991.
Wittgenstein, Ludwig. *Philosophical Occasions 1912–1951*. Oxford: Hackett, 1993.
Wittgenstein, Ludwig. Translated by Gertrude E. M. Anscombe. *Zettel*. Oxford: Blackwell, 1998.
Wittgenstein, Ludwig. *Tractatus Logico-Philosophicus*. Translated by D. F. Pears and B. F. McGuinness. London: Routledge, 2001.
Wittgenstein, Ludwig. *Blue Book*. Oxford: Blackwell, 2007.
Wittgenstein, Ludwig. *Philosophical Investigations*. Translated by Gertrude E. M. Anscombe. London: Wiley-Blackwell, 2009.

Wittgenstein, Ludwig, Waismann, Friedrich, and Gordon, Baker, eds. *The Voices of Wittgenstein. The Vienna Circle. Ludwig Wittgenstein and Friedrich Waismann.* London: Routledge, 2003.

Wolf, Susan. *Freedom within Reason*. New York: Oxford University Press, 1990.

World Health Organization. *The ICD-10 Classification of Mental and Behavioural Disorders: Clinical Descriptions and Diagnostic Guidelines*. Geneva: World Health Organization, 1992.

Articles

Ahrén, Jennie, Chiesa, Flaminia, Klinteberg, Britt A., and Koupil, Ilona. 'Psychosocial Determinants and Family Background in Anorexia Nervosa-Results from the Stockholm Birth Cohort Study'. *International Journal of Eating Disorders*, 45.3 (2012): 362–9.

Ahrén, Jennie C., Chiesa, Flaminia, Koupil, Ilona. Klinteberg, Magnusson, Cecilia, Dalman, Christina, and Goodman, Anna. 'We Are Family – Parents, Siblings, and Eating Disorders in a Prospective Total-Population Study of 250,000 Swedish Males and Females'. *International Journal of Eating Disorders*, 46.7 (2013): 693–700.

Arcelus, Jon, Witcomb, Gemma L., and Mitchell, Alex. 'Mortality Rates in Patients with Anorexia Nervosa and Other Eating Disorders. A Meta-Analysis of 36 Studies'. *Archives of General Psychiatry*, 68.7 (2011): 724–31.

Arcelus, Jon, Witcomb, Gemma L., Mitchell, Alex. 'Prevalence of Eating Disorders amongst Dancers: A Systematic Review and Meta-Analysis'. *European Eating Disorders Review*, 22.2 (2014): 92–101.

Attia, Evelyn. 'Anorexia Nervosa: Current Status and Future Directions'. *Annual Review of Medicine*, 61.1 (2010): 425–35.

Baxter, Helen. 'Religion and Eating Disorder'. *European Eating Disorders Review*, 9 (2001): 137–9.

Benson, Paul. 'Autonomy and Oppressive Socialization'. *Social Theory and Practice*, 17.3 (1991): 385–408.

Benson, Paul. 'Free Agent and Self-Worth'. *Journal of Philosophy*, 91.12 (1994): 656–7.

Benson, Paul. 'Narrative Self-Understanding and Relational Autonomy. Comments on Catriona Mackenzie and Jacqui Poltera, "'Narrative Integration, Fragmented Selves, and Autonomy" and Andrea C. Westlund "Rethinking Relation Autonomy"'. *Symposia on Gender, Race and Philosophy*, 7.1 (2011): 1–5.

Blinder, Barton J., Cumella, Edward J., and Sanathara, Visant A. 'Psychiatric Comorbidities of Female Inpatients with Eating Disorders'. *Psychosomatic Medicine*, 68.3 (2006): 454–62.

Boyle, Sam. 'How Should the Law Determine Capacity to Refuse Treatment for Anorexia?'. *International Journal of Law and Psychiatry*, 64 (2019): 250–9.

Bowden, Hanna. 'Is Anorexia Nervosa a Passion?'. *Philosophy, Psychiatry, & Psychology*, 20.4 (2013): 367–70.

Brecher, Robert. 'Why the Kantian Ideal Survives Medical Learning Curves, and Why It Matters'. *Journal of Medical Ethics*, 32.9 (2006): 511–12.

Brockmeyer, Timo, Holtforth, Martin Grosse, Bents, Hinrich, Kämmerer, Annette, Herzog, Wolfgang, and Friederich, Hans-Christoph. 'The Thinner the

Better: Self-Esteem and Low Body Weight in Anorexia Nervosa'. *Clinical Psychology and Psychotherapy*, 20.5 (2013): 294–300.

Broomfield, Catherine, Stedal, Kristin, Touyz, Stephen, and Rhodes, Paul. 'Labeling and Defining Severe and Enduring Anorexia Nervosa: A Systematic Review and Critical Analysis'. *International Journal of Eating Disorders*, 50.6 (2017): 611–23.

Brytek-Matera, Anna. 'Anorexia Nervosa among French Adolescent Females in Relation to Self-Esteem, Coping Strategies, Anger Expression and Anger Control'. *Archives of Psychiatry and Psychotherapy*, 4 (2007): 53–7.

Burke, Freddy, Maree, Higgins, and MacGinley, Maureen. '"I'll Do It on My Own, but I'm Never Alone": Lived Experience and Practitioner Perspectives of Autonomy in Longstanding and Severe Eating Disorder Treatment and Recovery – a Rapid Evidence Review'. *Journal of Eating Disorders* 12:208 (2024): 402–23.

Cave, Emma, and Tan, Jacinta. 'Severe and Enduring Anorexia Nervosa in the Court of Protection in England and Wales'. *International Journal of Mental Health and Capacity Law*, 23.17 (2017): 4–24.

Charland, Louis C., Hope, Tony, Stewart, Anne, and Tan, Jacinta. 'Anorexia Nervosa as a Passion'. *Philosophy, Psychiatry, & Psychology*, 20.4 (2013): 353–65.

Carter, Adam J., Kallestrup, Jesper, Palermos, Orestis S., and Pritchard, Duncan. 'Varieties of Externalism'. *Philosophical Issues*, 24.2 (2014): 63–109.

Christman, John. 'Autonomy and Personal History'. *Canadian Journal of Philosophy*, 21.1 (1991): 1–24.

Christman, John. 'Relational Autonomy, Liberal Individualism, and the Social Construction of Selves'. *Philosophical Studies*, 117.1/2 (2004): 143–64.

Clucas, Claudine. 'Understanding Self-Respect and Its Relationship to Self-Esteem'. *Personality and Social Psychology Bulletin*, 46.6 (2009): 1–17.

Conti, Janet E. 'Recovering Identity from Anorexia Nervosa: Women's Constructions of Their Experiences of Recovery from Anorexia Nervosa Over 10 Years'. *Journal of Constructivist Psychology*, 31.1 (2018): 72–94.

Conti, Janet, Rhodes, Paul, and Adams, Heather.'Listening in the Dark: Why We Need Stories of People Living with Severe and Enduring Anorexia Nervosa'. *Journal of Eating Disorders*, 4.33 (2016): 1–7.

Crisp, Arthur. 'Death, Survival And Recovery in Anorexia Nervosa: A Thirty Five Year Study'. *European Eating Disorders Review*, 14.3 (2006): 168–75.

Cudd, Ann E. 'Oppression by Choice'. *Journal of Social Philosophy*, 25.1 (1994): 22–44.

Dalla Grave, Rirccardo, El Ghoch, Marwan, Sartirana, Massimiliano, and Calugi, Simona. 'Cognitive Behavioral Therapy for Anorexia Nervosa: An Update'. *Current Psychiatry Reports*, 18.1 (2016): 1–18.

Davidson, Donald. 'Radical Interpretation'. *Dialectica*, 27.3/4 (1973): 313–28.

Diamond, Cora. 'Losing Your Concepts'. *Ethics*, 98.2 (1988): 255–77.

Dillon, Robin. S. 'Toward a Feminist Conception of Self-Respect'. *Hypatia*, 7.1 (1992): 52–69.

Domínguez-Rué, Emma. 'Sins of the Flesh: Anorexia, Eroticism and the Female Vampire in Bram Stoker's Dracula'. *Journal of Gender Studies*, 19.3 (2010): 297–308.

Draper, Heather. 'Anorexia Nervosa and Respecting a Refusal of Life-Prolonging Therapy: A Limited Justification'. *Bioethics*, 14.2 (2000): 120–33.

Dring, Greg. 'Anorexia Runs in Families: Is This due to Genes or the Family Environment?' *Journal of Family Therapy*, 37.1 (2015): 79–92.

Eddy, Kamryn T., Hennessey, Moira, and Thompson-Brenner, Heather. 'Eating Pathology in East African Women: The Role of Media Exposure and Globalization'. *Journal of Nervous and Mental Disease*, 195.3 (2007): 196–202.

Eisler, Ivan, Dare, Christopher, Hodes, Matthew, Russell, Gerald F., Dodge, Elizabeth, and Le Grange, Daniel. 'Family Therapy for Adolescent Anorexia Nervosa: The Results of a Controlled Comparison of Two Family Interventions'. *Journal of Child Psychology and Psychiatry, and Allied Disciplines*, 41.6 (2000): 727–36.

Esposito, Roberto, Cieri, Filippo, Di Giannantonio, Massimo, and Tartaro, Armando. 'The Role of Body Image and Self-Perception in Anorexia Nervosa: The Neuroimaging Perspective'. *Journal of Neuropsychology*, 12.1 (2016): 1–12.

Fairburn, Cristopher G., Cooper, Zafra, and Shafran, Roz. 'Cognitive Behaviour Therapy for Eating Disorders: A "Transdiagnostic" Theory and Treatment'. *Behaviour Research and Therapy*, 41.5 (2003): 509–28.

Fineman, Martha A. 'The Vulnerable Subject and the Responsive State'. *Emory Law Journal*, 60.2 (2010): 251–75.

Fitzpatrick, Kathleen K., and Lock, James D. 'Anorexia Nervosa'. *Journal of Shoulder and Elbow Surgery*, 20.6 (2011): 1008–15.

Foerde, Karin, Steinglass, Joanna E., Shohamy, Daphna, and Walsh, Timothy B. 'Neural Mechanisms Supporting Maladaptive Food Choices in Anorexia Nervosa'. *Nature Neuroscience*, 18.11 (2015): 1571–3.

Foot, Philippa. 'Does Moral Subjectivism Rest on a Mistake?'. *Oxford Journal of Legal Studies*, 15.1 (1995): 1–14.

Forcen, Fernando E. 'Anorexia Mirabilis: The Practice of Fasting by Saint Catherine of Siena in the Late Middle Ages'. *American Journal of Psychiatry*, 170.4 (2013): 370–1.

Freyenhagen, Fabian, and O'Shea, Tom. 'Hidden Substance: Mental Disorder as a Challenge to Normatively Neutral Accounts of Autonomy'. *International Journal of Law in Context*, 9.11 (2013): 53–70.

Giordano, Simona. 'Anorexia Nervosa and Its Moral Foundations'. *International Journal of Children's Rights*, 13.1–2 (2005): 149–60.

Giordano, Simona. 'Anorexia Nervosa: A Case for Exceptionalism in Ethical Decision Making'. *Philosophy, Psychiatry & Psychology*, 26.4 (2019): 315–31.

Goldman A. H. 'Reason Internalism'. *Philosophy and Phenomenological Research*, 71.3 (2005): 505–32.

Goodman, Alan, Heshmati, Amy, and Koupil, Ilona. 'Family History of Education Predicts Eating Disorders across Multiple Generations among 2 Million Swedish Males and Females'. *PLoS ONE*, 9.8 (2014): 1–9.

Gooldin, Sigal. 'Being Anorexic: Hunger, Subjectivity, and Embodied Morality'. *Medical Anthropology Quarterly*, 22.3 (2008): 274–96.

Govier, Trudy. 'Self-Trust, Autonomy, and Self-Esteem'. *Hypatia*, 8.1 (1993): 55–9.

Griffin, Joan M., and Berry, Elliot M. 'A Modern Day Holy Anorexia? Religious Language in Advertising and Anorexia Nervosa in the West'. *European Journal of Clinical Nutrition*, 57 (2003): 43–51.

Grisso, Thomas, Appelbaum, Paul S., and Hill-Fotouhi, Carolyn. 'The MacCAT-T: A Clinical Tool to Assess Patients' Capacities to Make Treatment Decisions'. *Psychiatric Services*, 48.11 (1997): 1415–19.

Gwizdek, Anna, Gwizdek, Katarzyna, and Koszowska, Agnieszka. 'Pro-Ana, Murderous Face of the Internet'. *Progress in Health Sciences*, 2.1 (2012): 158–61.

Halvorsen, Inger, and Heyerdahl, Sonja. 'Girls with Anorexia Nervosa as Young Adults: Personality, Self-Esteem, and Life Satisfaction'. *International Journal of Eating Disorders*, 39.4 (2006): 285–93.

Hay, Phillipa J., Touyz, Stephen, and Sud, Rishi. 'Treatment for Severe and Enduring Anorexia Nervosa: A Review'. *Australian and New Zealand Journal of Psychiatry*, 46.12 (2012): 1136–44.

Hay, Phillipa J., and Touyz, Stephen. 'Classification Challenges in the Field of Eating Disorders: Can Severe and Enduring Anorexia Nervosa Be Better Defined?'. *Journal of Eating Disorders*, 6.41 (2018): 1–3.

Hay, Phillipa J., and Touyz, Stephen. 'Treatment of Patients with Severe and Enduring Eating Disorders'. *Current Opinion in Psychiatry*, 28.6 (2015): 473–7.

Hope, Tony, Tan, Jacinta, Stewart, Anne, and Fitzpatrick, Ray. 'Anorexia Nervosa and the Language of Authenticity'. *Hastings Center Report*, 41.6 (2011): 19–29.

Hope, Tony, Tan, Jacinta, Stewart, Anne, and McMillan, John. 'Agency, Ambivalence and Authenticity: The Many Ways in Which Anorexia Nervosa Can Affect Autonomy'. *International Journal of Law in Context*, 9.1 (2013): 20–36.

Huline-Dickens, S. 'Anorexia Nervosa: Some Connections with the Religious Attitude'. *British Journal of Medical Psychology*, 73.1 (2000): 67–76.

Kakhi, Sara, and McCann, Jacinta. 'Anorexia Nervosa: Diagnosis, Risk Factors and Evidence-Based Treatments'. *Progress in Neurology and Psychiatry*, 20.6 (2016): 24–29c.

Karpowicz, Ewa, Skärsäter, Ingela, and Lauri, Nevonen. 'Self-Esteem in Patients Treated for Anorexia Nervosa'. *International Journal of Mental Health Nursing*, 18.5 (2009): 318–25.

Kästner, Denise, Löwe, Bernd, and Gumz, Antje. 'The Role of Self-Esteem in the Treatment of Patients with Anorexia Nervosa – a Systematic Review and Meta-Analysis'. *International Journal of Eating Disorders*, 52.2 (2019): 101–16.

Keel, Pamela K., and Brown, Tiffany A. 'Update on Course and Outcome in Eating Disorders'. *International Journal of Eating Disorders*, 43.3 (2010): 195–204.

Khader, Serene. 'Beyond Autonomy Fetishism: Affiliation with Autonomy in Women's Empowerment'. *Journal of Human Development and Capabilities*, 17.1 (2016): 125–39.

Kipman, Amélie, Kipman, Amélie, Gorwood, Philip, Mouren-Siméoni, Marie-Christine, and Adès, Jacques. 'Genetic Factors in Anorexia Nervosa'. *European Psychiatry*, 14.4 (1999): 189–98.

Kong, Camillia. 'Beyond the Balancing Scales: The Importance of Prejudice and Dialogue in A Local Authority v E et al.' *Child and Family Law Quarterly*, 26.2 (2014): 216–36.

Ip, Eric C. 'Anorexia Nervosa, Advance Directives, and the Law: A British Perspective'. *Bioethics*, 33.8 (2019): 931–6.

Jamieson, Sacha K., Tan, Jacinta, Piekunka, Kym, Calvert, Shannon, and Stephen, Anderson. 'Navigating the Ethical Complexities of Severe and Enduring Eating Disorders: Tools for Critically Reflective Practice and Collaborative Decision-Making'. *Journal of Eating Disorders* 12.134 (2024): 1–17.

LaMarre, Andrea, Tan, Jacinta, Piekunka, Kym, Calvert, Shannon, and Anderson, Stephen. 'An Open Invitation to Productive Conversations about Feminism and the Spectrum of Eating Disorders (Part 1): Basic Principles of Feminist Approaches'. *Journal of Eating Disorders*, 10.54 (2022): 1–12.

Lampard, Amy M., Tasca, Giorgio A., Balfour, Louise, and Bissada, Hany. 'An Evaluation of the Transdiagnostic Cognitive-Behavioural Model of Eating Disorders'. *European Eating Disorders Review*, 21.2 (2013): 99–107.

Le Grange, Daniel, Telch F., Christy, and Tibbs, Jason. 'Eating Attitudes and Behaviors in 1435 South African Caucasian and Non-Caucasian College Students'. *American Journal of Psychiatry*, 155.2 (1998): 250–4.

Lindberg, Lene, and Hjern, Andres. 'Risk Factors for Anorexia Nervosa: A National Cohort Study'. *International Journal of Eating Disorders*, 34.4 (2003): 397–408.

Lindstedt, Katarina, Kjellin, Lars, and Gustafsson, Sanna A. 'Adolescent with Full or Subthreshold Anorexia Nervosa in a Naturalistic Sample – Characteristics and Treatment Outcome'. *Journal of Eating Disorders*, 5.4 (2017): 1–13.

Martin, Wayne, Freyenhagen, Fabian, Hall, Elizabeth, O'Shea, Tom, Szerletics, Antal, and Ashley, Vivienne. 'An Unblinkered View of Best Interests'. *BMJ*, 345 (Online) (2012).

McClelland, Lisa, and Crisp, Arthur. 'Anorexia Nervosa and Social Class'. *International Journal of Eating Disorders*, 29.2 (2001): 150–6.

Mendhekar, Dattatreya N., Arora, Kavita, Lohia, Deep, Aggarwal, Ashish, and Jiloha, Ram C. 'Anorexia Nervosa: An Indian Perspective'. *National Medical Journal of India*, 22.4 (2009): 181–2.

Meyers, Diana. 'Feminism and Women's Autonomy: The Challenge of Female Genital Cutting'. *Metaphilosophy*, 31.5 (2000): 469–91.

Murray, Stuart B., Nagata, Jason M., Griffiths, Scott, Calzo, Jerel P., Brown, Tiffany A., Mitchison, Deborah, Blashill, Aaron J., and Mond, Jonathan M. 'The Enigma of Male Eating Disorders: A Critical Review and Synthesis'. *Clinical Psychology Review*, 57 (2017): 1–11.

Nasser, Mervat. 'Eating Disorders across Cultures'. *Psychiatry*, 6.9 (2009): 347–50.

Nishizono-Maher, Aya. 'Eating Disorders in Japan: Finding the Right Context'. *Psychiatry and Clinical Neurosciences*, 52 Suppl. (1998): 320–3.

Norman, Richard. 'Practical Reasons and the Redundancy of Motives'. *Ethical Theory and Moral practice*, 4 (2001): 3–22.

Norris, Sophie C., Gleaves, David H., and Hutchinson, Amanda D. 'Anorexia Nervosa and Perfectionism: A Meta-Analysis'. *International Journal of Eating Disorders*, 52.3 (2019): 219–29.

Nussbaum, Martha. 'Symposium on Amartya Sen's Philosophy: 5 Adaptive Preferences and Women's Options'. *Economics and Philosophy*, 17.1 (2001): 67–88.

Nussbaum, Martha. 'Political Liberalism and Respect: A Response to Linda Barclay'. *SATS: Nordic Journal of Philosophy*, 4.2 (2003): 25–44.

Oldershaw, Anna, Startup, Helen, and Lavender, Tony. 'Anorexia Nervosa and a Lost Emotional Self: A Psychological Formulation of the Development, Maintenance, and Treatment of Anorexia Nervosa'. *Frontiers of Psychology*, 10.219 (2019): 1–22.

Oshana, Marina. 'Personal Autonomy and Society'. *Canadian Journal of Philosophy*, 29.1 (1998): 81–102.

Owen, Gareth S., Freyenhagen, Fabian, Richardson, Genevera, and Hotopf, Matthew. 'Mental Capacity and Decisional Autonomy: An Interdisciplinary Challenge'. *Inquiry*, 52.1 (2009): 79–107.

Owen, Gareth, Martin, Wayne, and Gergel, Tania. 'Misevaluating the Future: Affective Disorder and Decision-Making Capacity for Treatment – a Temporal Understanding'. *Psychopathology*, 51.6 (2018): 371–9.

Park, Rebecca J., Singh, Ilina, Pike, Alexandra C., and Tan, Jacinta O. A. 'Deep Brain Stimulation in Anorexia Nervosa: Hope for the Hopeless or Exploitation of the Vulnerable? The Oxford Neuroethics Gold Standard Framework'. *Frontiers in Psychiatry*, 8.44 (2017): 1–10.

Patrone, Daniel. 'Disfigured Anatomies and Imperfect Analogies: Body Integrity Identity Disorder and the Supposed Right to Self-Demanded Amputation of Healthy Body Parts'. *Journal of Medical Ethics*, 35.9 (2009): 541–5.

Pearce, John. M. S. 'Richard Morton: Origins of Anorexia Nervosa'. *European Neurology*, 52.4 (2004): 191–2.

Pennesi, Jamie-Lee, and Wade, Trace D. 'A Systematic Review of the Existing Models of Disordered Eating: Do They Inform the Development of Effective Interventions?'. *Clinical Psychology Review*, 43 (2016): 175–92.

Phillipou, Andrea, Rossell, Susan L., Gurvich, Caroline, Jonathan Castle, David, Troje, Nikolaus F., and Abel, Larry A. 'Body Image in Anorexia Nervosa: Body Size Estimation Utilising a Biological Motion Task and Eyetracking'. *European Eating Disorders Review*, 24.2 (2016): 131–8.

Pike, Kathleen M., Hilbert, Anja, Wilfley, Denise E., Fairburn, Christopher G., Dohm, Faith-Anne, Walsh, Bernard T., and Striegel-Moore, Ruth H. 'Toward an Understanding of Risk Factors for Anorexia Nervosa: A Case-Control Study'. *Psychological Medicine*, 38.10 (2008): 1443–53.

Pike, Kathleen M., and Dunne, Patricia E. 'The Rise of Eating Disorders in Asia: A Review'. *Journal of Eating Disorders*, 3.1 (2015): 33.

Pittock, Alexandra. 'How Are Anorexia Nervosa and Spirituality Connected, and What Implications Does This Have for Treatment?'. *Royal College of Psychiatrists*, 1 (2014): 1–14.

Polivy, Janet, and Herman, C. Peter. 'Causes of Eating Disorders'. *Annual Review of Psychology*, 53 (2002): 187–213.

Preti, Antonio, Usai, Ambra, Miotto, Paola, Petretto, Donatella R., and Masala, Carmelo. 'Eating Disorders among Professional Fashion Models'. *Psychiatry Research*, 159.1–2 (2008): 86–94.

Rodhe, Paul, Stice, Eric, and Marti, Nathan C. 'Development and Predictive Effects of Eating Disorder Risk Factors during Adolescence: Implication for Prevention Efforts'. *International Journal of Eating Disorders*, 48.2 (2015): 187–98.

Robinson, Paul, Kukucska, Roza, Guidetti, Giulia, and Leavey, Gerard. 'Severe and Enduring Anorexia Nervosa (SEED-AN): A Qualitative Study of Patients with 20+ Years of Anorexia Nervosa'. *European Eating Disorder Review*, 23.4 (2015): 318–26.

Ryan, Christopher J. 'Out on a Limb: The Ethical Management of Body Integrity Identity Disorder'. *Neuroethics*, 2.1 (2009): 21–33.

Schauenburg, Henning, Friederich, Hans-Cristoph, Wild, Beate, and Zipfel, Stephan. 'Focal Psychodynamic Psychotherapy of Anorexia Nervosa: A Treatment Manual'. *Psychotherapeut*, 54.4 (2009): 270–80.

Schott, Nicole D., and Langan, Debra. 'Pro-Anorexia/Bulimia Censorship and Public Service Announcements: The Price of Controlling Women'. *Media, Culture & Society*, 37.8 (2015): 1158–73.

Schreyer, Colleen, Coughlin, Janelle W., Makhzoumi, Saniha H., Redgrave, Graham W., Hansen, Jennifer L., and Guarda, Angela S. 'Perceived Coercion in Inpatients with Anorexia Nervosa: Associations with Illness Severity and Hospital Course'. *International Journal of Eating Disorders*, 49.4 (2016): 107–412.

Shade, Leslie R. 'Weborexics: The Ethical Issues Surrounding Pro-Ana Websites'. *ACM SIGCAS Computers and Society*, 33.4 (2003): 2.

Smink, Frédérique R. E., van Hoeken, Daphne, and Hoek, Hans W. 'Epidemiology of Eating Disorders: Incidence, Prevalence and Mortality Rates'. *Current Psychiatry Reports*, 14.4 (2012): 406–14.

Sobel, David. 'Explanation, Internalism, and Reasons for Action'. *Social Philosophy and Policy*, 18.2 (2001): 218–35.

Spear, Andrew D. 'Epistemic Dimension of Gaslighting: Peer-Disagreement, Self-Trust, and Epistemic Injustice'. *Inquiry: An Interdisciplinary Journal of Philosophy*, 1 (2019): 1–24.

Strife, Samantha R., and Rickard, Kathryn. 'The Conceptualization of Anorexia: The Pro-Ana Perspective'. *Affilia*, 26.2 (2011): 213–17.

Sullivan, Laura S., and Niker, Fay. 'Relational Autonomy, Paternalism, and Maternalism'. *Ethical Theory and Moral Practice*, 21.3 (2018): 649–67.

Superson, Anita. 'Deformed Desires and Informed Desire Tests'. *Hypatia*, 20.4 (2005): 109–26.

Tafarodi, Robin. W., and Swann, William B. Jr. 'Self-Liking and Self-Competence as Dimension of Global Self-Esteem: Initial Validation of a Measure'. *Journal of Personality Assessment*, 65.2 (2010): 322–42.

Tan, Jacinta O. A, Hope, Tony, and Stewart, Anne. 'Anorexia Nervosa and Personal Identity: The Accounts of Patients and Their Parents'. *International Journal of Law and Psychiatry*, 26.5 (2003): 533–48.

Tan, Jacinta O. A, Hope, Tony, Stewart, Anne, and Fitzpatrick, Raymond. 'Control and Compulsory Treatment in Anorexia Nervosa: The Views of Patients and Parents'. *International Journal of Law and Psychiatry*, 26.6 (2003): 627–45.

Tan, Jacinta O. A, Hope, Tan, and Stewart, Anne. 'Competence to Refuse Treatment in Anorexia Nervosa'. *International Journal of Law and Psychiatry*, 26.6 (2003): 697–707.

Tan, Jacinta O. A, Hope, Tony, Stewart, Anne, and Fitzpatrick, Raymond. 'Competence to Make Treatment Decisions in Anorexia Nervosa: Thinking Processes and Values'. *Philosophy, Psychiatry, & Psychology*, 13 (2006): 267–82.

Tan, Jacinta O. A, Stewart, Anne, Fitzpatrick, Raymond, and Hope, Tony. 'Attitudes of Patients with Anorexia Nervosa to Compulsory Treatment and Coercion'. *International Journal of Law and Psychiatry*, 33.1 (2010): 13–19.

Tan, Jacinta O. A, Karim, Syahirah, Lee, Huei Y., and Yen, Goh L. 'Cultural and Ethical Issues in the Treatment of Eating Disorders in Singapore'. *Asian Bioethics Review*, 5.1 (2013): 40–55.

Touyz, Stephen, and Hay, Philipa. 'Severe and Enduring Anorexia Nervosa (SEAN): in Search of a New Paradigm'. *Journal of Eating Disorders*, 3.26 (2015): 1–3.

Touyz, Stephen, Aouad, Phillip, Carney, Terry, Ong, Shu H., Yager, Joel, Newton, Richard, Hay, Phillipa, Maguire, Sarah, and Bryant, Emma. 'Clinical, Legal and Ethical Implications of Coercion and Compulsory Treatment in Eating Disorders: Do Rapid Review Findings Identify Clear Answers or More Muddy Waters?'. *Journal of Eating Disorders*, 12.163 (2024): 1–16.

Walters, Ellen E., and Kendler, Kenneth S. 'Anorexia Nervosa and Anorexic-like Syndromes in a Population-Based Female Twin Sample'. *American Journal of Psychiatry*, 152.1 (1995): 64–71.

Wang, Daniel W. L. 'Mental Capacity Act, Anorexia Nervosa and the Choice Between Life-Prolonging Treatment and Palliative Care: A NHS Foundation Trust v Ms X'. *Modern Law Review*, 78.5 (2015): 871–82.

Ward, Anne, Ramsay, Rosalind, Russell, Gerald, and Treasure, Janet. 'Follow-Up Mortality Study of Compulsory Treated Patients with Anorexia Nervosa'. *International Journal of Eating Disorders*, 48.7 (2015): 860–5.

Wardle, Jane, Rosato, Marco S., Desousa, Avinash, and Cotrufo, Paolo. 'Culture and Body Image: Body Perception and Weight Concern in Young Asian and Caucasian British Women'. *Journal of Community & Applied Social Psychology*, 3.3 (1993): 173–81.

Weinberg, Cybelle. 'From the Ascetic Ideal to the Esthetic Ideal: The Historical Evolution of Anorexia Nervosa'. *Revista Latinoamericana de Psicopatologia Fundamental*, 13.2 (2010): 224–37.

Westlund, Andrea C. 'Selflessness and Responsibility for Self: The Implications of Deference for Autonomy, Shared Agency and Love'. *ProQuest Dissertations and Theses* (2001): 483–523.

Westlund, Andrea C. 'Rethinking Relational Autonomy'. *Hypatia*, 24.4 (2009): 26–49.

Young, Kate, Fisher, Jane, and Kirkman, Maggie. "Do Mad People Get Endo or Does Endo Make You Mad?': Clinicians' Discoursive Construction of Medicine and Women with Endometriosis'. *Feminism and Psychology*, 29.3 (2019): 337–56.

Zeeck, Almut, Herpertz-Dahlmann, Beate, Friederich, Hans-Christoph, Brockmeyer, Timo, Resmark, Gaby, Hagenah, Ulrich, Ehrlich, Stefan, Cuntz, Ulrich, Zipfel, Stephan, and Hartmann, Armin. 'Psychotherapeutic Treatment for Anorexia Nervosa: A Systematic Review and Network Meta-Analysis'. *Frontiers in Psychiatry*, 9.158 (2018): 1–14.

Zipfel, Stephan, Giel, Katrin E., Bulik, Cynthia M., Hay, Phillipa, and Schmidt, Ulrike. 'Anorexia Nervosa: Aetiology, Assessment and Treatment'. *Lancet Psychiatry*, 2.12 (2015): 1099–111.

Acts of parliament, sentences of the court of protection, conventions

A Local Authority v E (2012) EWCOP 1639

A NHS Foundation Trust v MS X (2014) EWCOP 35

L. Donaldson, Re T (Adult) (1992), 4 All ER 649

Mental Capacity Act 2005

Mental Health Act 1983

Mental Health Act Commission (MHAC), *Guidance on the Treatment of Anorexia under the Mental Health Act 1983*, London, HMSO (1997)

Re T (An Adult) Consent to Treatment (1992) 4 All ER 649 (CA).

Sidaway (Appellant) *v Bethlem Royal Hospital and the Maudesley Hospital Health Authority et al* (1985) 1 All ER 643

Documentaries and YouTube video

Special Books by Special Kids. 'Battling Chronic Anorexia for Over a Decade (But Still Fighting for Recovery)'. YouTube video, posted 2 November 2018. https://www.youtube.com/watch?v=NOoNYdhYOWY.

EssexAutonomyProject. 'Fabian Freyenhagen – the Philosophical Terrain'. YouTube video, posted 26 April 2012. https://www.youtube.com/watch?v=F4-B6JH91dM&t=989s.
Louis Theroux. 'Louis Theroux: Talking to Anorexia'. BBC documentary, BBC, 2017.

Websites, blogs, newspapers

Alexander J. 'Severe and Enduring Anorexia Nervosa – Should We Even Give Up?', *Diary Healer*, Web Blog, 12 September 2017. https://www.thediaryhealer.com/2017/09/12/severe-and-enduring-anorexia-nervosa-should-we-ever-give-up.
Pro Ana Goddess, *Tips & Tricks*. Web Blog. https://proanagoddess.wordpress.com/tips-tricks-2.
Schmidt, S. 'Anorexic Woman Weighing 69 Pounds Has a Right to Starve, Court Rules'. *Washington Post*, 22 November 2016. https://www.washingtonpost.com/gdpr-consent/?next_url=https%3a%2f%2fwww.washingtonpost.com%2fnews%2fmorning-mix%2fwp%2f2016%2f11%2f22%2fanorexic-woman-weighing-69-pounds-has-a-right-to-starve-court-rules%2f.
SonsofAna. *Ana Has a Set of 10 Commandments – Follow Them*. Web Blog. https://sonsofana.weebly.com/anas-commandments.html.
SonsofAna. *Read It Live It*. Web Blog. https://sonsofana.weebly.com/creeds-and-mantras.html.
'Surgeon Defends Amputation'. *BBC News*, 31 January 2000. http://news.bbc.co.uk/1/hi/scotland/625680.stm.
Whoreomel. *Hiding your ED*. Web Blog. https://whoreomel.wixsite.com/proana/hiding-your-ed.

Index

A Local Authority v E (2012) 38–40
A NHS Foundation Trust v Ms X (2014) 40–3
affect, affective dimension 17–25, 33–35, 37–49, 79–82, 118–120
agency 3–14, 53–62, 66–9, 72–90, 106–12, 117–23, 127, 139–42
anorexia nervosa
  clinical features 1–2, 15–17
  historical, religious interpretations 16–7, 29–32
  identity, authenticity and anorexia 17–35, 115–26, 139–41
  neurological studies 42–3
  risk factors, sociocultural context 28–32
  severe and enduring anorexia 135–8
  treatment, recovery 15–7, 25–7, 126–38
  treatment refusal, legal status 1–6, 37–49, 115–38
autonomy
  in anorexia 1–5, 15–35, 37–49, 115–38, 139–42
  concept of 1–6, 32–5, 44–49, 51–69, 71–90, 91–114, 115–18, 125–38, 139–42
  conditions for exercise of 91–114, 115–38, 139–42
  dialogical conception 3–4, 7–14, 61, 68, 91–114, 124–38, 139–42
  feminism and autonomy 28–32, 71–90
  monological 65–9, 84–90, 94–5, 99–100, 114–18, 140–2
  liberal and individualist models 1–4, 51–69, 71–80, 115–24
  relational accounts 6–13, 71–90, 91–114, 115–38
  weak substantivism 9–13, 73–5, 77, 86, 91–3, 104–6, 111, 116–18

background, normative 54–6, 94–114, 139–42
best interests 42–5, 115–38
body image 1–3, 17, 42
body perception 16, 42
Bruch, Hilde 21–2

capacity, decision-making, *see* decisional capacity
care, relational 71–90, 115–38
Christman, John 77–9, 87–9, 105–6
Code, Lorraine 72
Convention on the Rights of Persons with Disabilities (CRPD) 38–40
control, sense of 18–27, 118–26

decisional capacity 3–6, 37–49, 51–69, 115–38, 139–42
dialogical answerability 8–14, 48–9, 91–114, 115–38, 139–42
dialogical autonomy, *see* autonomy, dialogical conception
dialogical responsibility 115–38
Double Axis theory 47–9, 91–3

eating disorders (general) 15–17
egosyntonicity 13–14, 18–25, 57–62, 118–26
externalism of reasons 51–6, 62–5

force-feeding 4–6, 37–49, 115–38
functional test of capacity 37–49, 58–61

Giordano, Simona 4–6, 33–5, 41–49, 56–8, 65–9, 115–16, 130, 137
global and local autonomy 104–6

identity (personal, anorexic) 18–25, 25–35, 91–114, 139–42
internalism of reasons 51–69
intervention, paternalism 44–5, 82, 89–90, 115–18, 134–8

language, private and public 94–104
liberalism 51–69, 71–72, 80, 139–40

MacArthur Competence Assessment Tool for Treatment (MacCATT) 38–9
Mackenzie, Catriona 72, 75–82, 89–90, 106–7, 114
MacIntyre, Alasdair 80–1, 91–4
mental capacity 1–14, 37–49, 52–3, 59–60, 115–38
Mental Capacity Act 2005 (MCA) 3–11, 37–41, 52–3, 140–2
Mental Health Act 1983 (MHA) 39–40
Meyers, Diana 47–8, 65–69, 91–3, 140

normativity, value-neutrality and value-ladenness, *see* value-neutrality

oppression 72–93, 113–14, 127–35

paternalism 62–5, 89–90, 115–18
private language argument 95–103
pro-ana websites and online communities 22–3, 27

reasons
  and autonomy 51–69
  external, *see* externalism of reasons
  internal, *see* internalism of reasons
recognition 106–14
relational autonomy, *see* autonomy, relational accounts
relational responsibility 115–18, 140–1

self-knowledge 91–104, 139–42
self-respect 107–8, 121–2
self-trust 118–26
self-worth and self-esteem 106–26
severe and enduring anorexia nervosa (SEAN), *see* anorexia, severe enduring anorexia

Taylor, Charles 7–13, 65–7, 85, 92–9, 139–42
treatment refusal, anorexia 1–5, 37–49, 115–38

value-neutrality 1–14, 45–9, 51–4, 65–9, 82–7, 91–3, 115–18, 140
vulnerability
  and autonomy 79–82, 86–90, 139–41
  inherent and situational 80–2, 108, 122

Westlund, Andrea 68, 110
Williams, Bernard 52–6
Wittgenstein, Ludwig 97–104

www.ingramcontent.com/pod-product-compliance
Ingram Content Group UK Ltd.
Pitfield, Milton Keynes, MK11 3LW, UK
UKHW020816290926
15470UKWH00003B/1194

9 781350 611665